LILAC

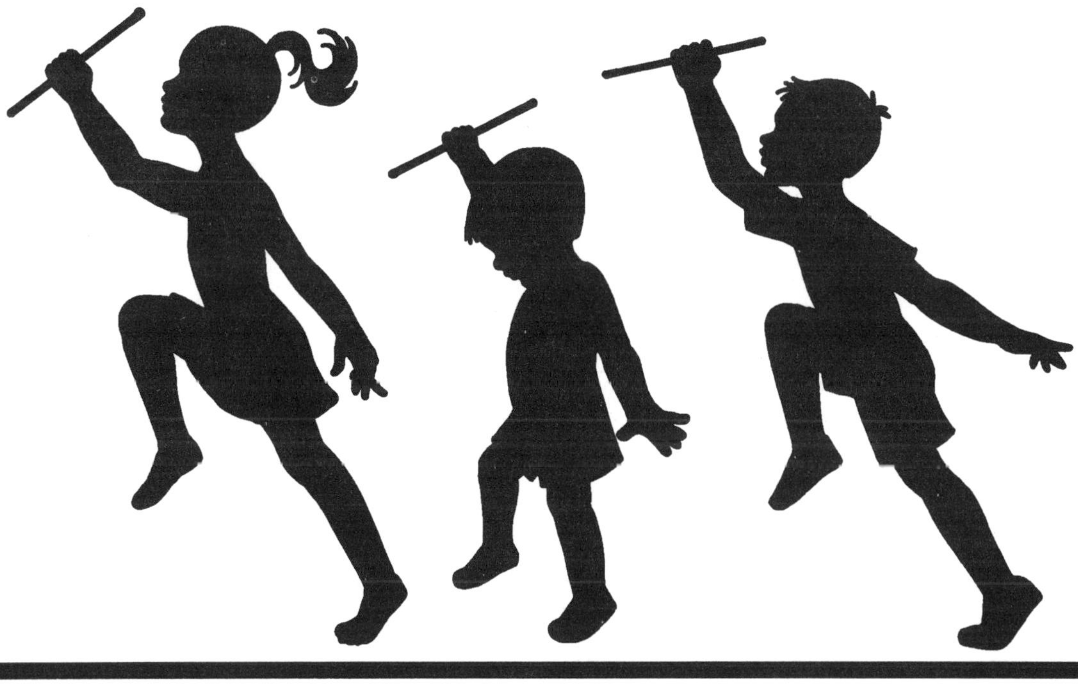

LESSONS FOR INCLUSIVE LANGUAGE ACTIVITIES IN THE CLASSROOM

Gail Raymond & Aileen C. Lau-Dickinson

The Speech Bin

Dedication

We are grateful to the staff of the Child Development Division,
Health and Human Services Finance Commission,
for their support in the development of this curriculum.
Our thanks go to the teachers and children of the Centers
who included our activities in their curriculum.
We especially appreciate the efforts of Dottie Garvey and Carolyn Durrell
for their encouragement and direction.
A special thanks goes to Lorin Anderson, Garrett Mandeville, and
Gay Clement-Atkinson for their suggestions and guidance.
We are grateful to the following teachers and graduate students for their help:
Netra Van Tassell, Mary Ringer, Beth M. Hui, Muff Lyons, Ann Cuddy,
Anita Grossman, Martha McCullough, Bonnie Chambers, Dottie Green, Evelyn Monroe,
Ray Roberts, Addie McAlister, Janet West, Barbara Luce, Allyn Brunner
Holly Brunner, Vicki Cooney, Lynne Perry, and Dana Winn.
Finally, we appreciate our families for
understanding our commitment to the project.

The Speech Bin, Inc.
1965 Twenty-Fifth Avenue
Vero Beach, Florida 32960

ISBN 0-937857-71-8
Catalog Number 1428

Printed in the United States of America

Table of Contents

Introduction

Many preschool children with speech-language delays or communication disorders are enrolled in programs, such as day care, child development classes, Headstart, and classes for three- to five-year-olds. These children perform best when they participate with their peers in programs that provide a natural setting in which language is used to send messages, give information, and ask questions. Language experiences should emphasize interacting with people, exchanging information, and learning language skills that will enhance future academic achievement.

In successful intervention programs language is taught through everyday routines in a natural way (Hart, and Rogers-Warren, 1978). More direct teaching approaches use language activities to help preschool children achieve sequenced language objectives (Engleman and Carmine, 1990). Both direct and naturalistic teaching approaches have strengths and weaknesses (Cole and Dale, 1986; McCormick and Schiefelbusch, 1990).

Lessons for Inclusive Language Activities in the Classroom (LILAC) provides a comprehensive guide to using both naturalistic and direct approaches to language development. It gives young students a wealth of opportunities to use language to request materials, describe activities, ask questions, and interact with others. These language activities help children improve skills in semantics, syntax, and receptive language. They can be used in direct teaching approaches or in a more naturalistic approach that stimulates oral language mastery through everyday routines.

Oral language mastery is critical for later success in reading and writing (Valencia, Pearson, Peters, and Wilson, 1989). Oral language, reading, and writing develop interdependently between the ages of three and eight. *LILAC* provides early childhood professionals, such as teachers and speech-language pathologists, with sequenced, hierarchical language activities that not only foster spoken language but link language to later reading and writing. Although these activities are appropriate for all children in preschool settings, they focus on specific skills needed by children with language delays.

LILAC includes more than 150 sequential activities based on established language skills. The language activities, appropriate for three- through five-year-old developmental levels, are identified as Levels A through E. Each Level contains five language areas:

- Vocabulary
- Concepts
- Sentences
- Stories
- Listening

Each activity includes an instructional objective and materials needed. Nearly all materials suggested are readily available in the typical preschool classroom. Many activities also include illustrations.

The *LILAC* program provides a series of lessons to facilitate expressive and receptive language development of preschoolers. It can be used with all preschool children because the scope and sequence of its activities are based on normal language acquisition. However, activities are especially useful for children who are at risk for later school failure because the emphasis is on language skills required for future success in reading.

LILAC includes a Language Scope and Sequence chart with objectives for each of the five language areas. They may be used as objectives in individualized educational or intervention programs. The program also has a Skills Check Chart that can be used as an informal screening tool to assist in determining a child's language level upon entrance into a program and to assess children's subsequent progress toward language goals.

LILAC is a condensed version of a longer, more detailed language program, the *DAISEY Program* (Lau and Raymond, 1993). *DAISEY* includes a two-stage assessment program, an instructional program, and 150 home activities for young children at risk for school success. It is not a curriculum in itself but is used to supplement curricula used in early childhood programs. It is active, creative, easy to use, and adaptable. It provides ongoing informal assessment and allows for children's individual differences and their special needs.

Who Should Use *LILAC*

Activities can be implemented by classroom teachers, speech-language pathologists, occupational therapists, paraprofessionals, volunteers, and parents and other family members at home. Speech-language pathologists and teachers may expand activities based on children's individual needs. Complete and detailed instructions are included, making activities easy to read and follow with minimal preparation.

Involving parents is critical to the success of any early childhood program. Parents may not think of themselves as teachers and need encouragement to recognize their importance in this critical role. Speech-language pathologists and other professionals should ensure parents know how language develops and how vital they are in the process (Andrews, 1986). This resource book includes activities and pictures that also can be used effectively by parents with their children at home. These home learning activities can give the parent both specific information about language and activities that are fun for both the child and the parent. Sample letters to parents are also included.

Summary

LILAC provides easy-to-implement activities for twenty-five developmental and sequential language objectives. This program is for all children, but it is particularly useful for language-delayed preschoolers. It can be easily implemented by paraprofessionals working closely with a classroom teacher or speech-language pathologist. Each activity is flexible and allows children to be creative and self-directive. Activities also may be presented in a direct manner with the leader presenting instructions in a clear and simple way.

How to Use *LILAC* and Implement Its Activities

A. Before teaching begins:

- Determine instructional level (A-E) appropriate for the children through evaluation or informal assessment. Children may be screened using the Skills Check Chart provided.

- Form small groups of children based on their functional level (A-E). Recommended group size is five to eight children (individual instruction may also be appropriate).

B. Before each activity session:

- Read though the day's activity.
- Make copies of illustrations that accompany the activity.
- Gather other materials.
- Be sure each child has a notebook or folder to keep any completed activities.

C. During the activity:

- Introduce the activity to the children. (Most activities can be introduced sitting on the floor to allow for freedom of movement.)
- Be sure each child has opportunity to participate in the group.
- Remember that the activities are meant to be active and fun.
- Encourage each child to gain experience with oral language.
- Give each child plenty of time to respond to the expectations of the activity.
- Allow children to be creative and develop their own ideas triggered by each activity.

D. Following each series of activities:

- Assess each child's progress, using the Skills Check provided.
- When a child masters an objective, enter date on the individual child's Skill Check Chart (kept on file).

Examples of Letters to Parents

Letter 1

Dear Parent:

We are so happy to have Lamar in our class this year. You are his most important teacher, and we are eager to work with you.

We are particularly interested in helping him to learn concepts to get him ready for school, such as learning counting and colors. We will work on language through activities, such as building vocabulary, telling stories, talking in sentences, and learning to follow directions.

We are looking forward to getting to know you. We hope you will visit our classroom often and encourage you to volunteer your time to assist with our daily activities.

Each week we will send home activity sheets for you to do with your child. The activities are simple and fun. They *will* help your child get ready to learn more advanced things. Please send us a note when you finish the activity and share your comments with us.

We are looking forward to a great year! I will call you soon to talk with you about your child.

Sincerely,

Letter 2

Dear Ms. Bowers:

We have enjoyed getting to know your daughter, Emily, during the past six weeks. She has been a pleasure to have in our class. She loves to play at the water table and in the housekeeping center.

As you know, we have worked on many language activities. She has learned to tell the function of her body parts, follow simple directions, and tell a simple story using complete sentences.

Thank you for returning the activity sheets each week with your comments. You have helped her a great deal. I hope that you can visit our class soon and participate in our activities.

Sincerely,

About the Authors

Gail I. Raymond, Associate Professor of Special Education, Department of Educational Psychology, University of South Carolina, and Aileen C. Lau-Dickinson, Adjunct Professor of Special Education, University of South Carolina, Columbia and Beaufort, are co-authors of *LILAC: Lessons for Inclusive Language Activities in the Classroom.* They have also developed an early childhood program, *Developmental Assessment and Instruction for Success in the Early Years (DAISEY).* Raymond and Aileen Lau-Dickinson received the 1991 Partnership in Education Award from Richland County School District-Two for their work with the *DAISEY Program* in Pontiac and Bethel-Hanbury Elementary Schools, Columbia, South Carolina.

Raymond earned the bachelor of arts in elementary education from Longwood College (Farmville, Virginia) and the master of education in counselor education and doctorate in education at University of South Carolina. She taught three years at University of New Orleans and has been a member of the faculty of College of Education, University of South Carolina, for twenty-two years. She has taught courses in educational assessment, education procedures, learning disabilities, and early childhood special education; directed internships with doctoral students and practica with doctoral and master's students. Through her teaching, in-service training, and consultation in school districts with regular and special education teachers she has helped educators understand the needs of students with mild disabilities and develop strategies to include these children in regular classrooms.

Raymond founded the Educational Services Clinic, Special Education, at the University of South Carolina as a training program in assessment procedures for graduate students. She has Raymond has served as the Clinic's Director for the past twenty years. She has been director of three grants in personnel preparation funded by United States Department of Education. She has also directed one foundation grant and seven projects funded by state grants from Department of Education, Health and Human Service Finance Commission, and Commission of Higher Education.

Aileen Lau-Dickinson earned her bachelor of arts in speech education at Northwestern University, master of science in speech-language pathology at University of Michigan, and doctorate of education in special education from University of South Carolina. She has worked as speech-language pathologist in a variety of clinical settings. She served as Director of Clinical Services at St. Nicholas Speech and Hearing Clinic, Greenwood, South Carolina (which she founded), Detroit Speech and Hearing Clinic, Walter E. Fernald State School, and Midlands Center for the Retarded; she was previously state coordinator for developmental centers in Massachusetts. She is a frequent presenter at seminars, workshops, and state and national meetings.

She teaches courses in language impairment in children, special education, early childhood special education, educational assessment, and early childhood special education procedures. She is a consultant in assistive technology and communication disorders to school districts and provides clinical services in speech-language pathology and assistive technology for community residential centers for Department for Disabilities and Special Needs and for Early Intervention Program, Naval Hospital, Beaufort.

Lau-Dickinson holds the Certificate of Clinical Competence in Speech-Language Pathology of American Speech-Language-Hearing Association and is a Fellow of the ASHA. She was awarded the Honors of South Carolina Speech-Language-Hearing Association and served as president of that organization. Other honors include Distinguished Service Award, Sturbridge (Massachusetts) Chamber of Commerce; Career Woman of the Year, Business and Professional Women of Greenwood; Service to Mankind Award, Greenwood Sertoma Club; and Greenwood United Way's Volunteer of the Year. Among her publications are *Curriculum and Resource Guide for Special Needs Students,* Massachusetts Department of Mental Retardation (1975), *Total Communication Program* (1979), and as co-author with Gail I. Raymond, the *DAISEY Program (1993).*

References

Anderson, L. Developmental assessment and instruction for success in the early years (DAISEY): Technical manual. Columbia, SC: Daisey Associates, 1987.

Andrews, A.B. *Promoting parent involvement: A handbook for child development centers.* Columbia, SC: University of South Carolina, 1986.

Bayley, N. *Bayley scales of infant development.* New York: Psychological Corporation, 1969.

Belgau, F.A. and Basden, B.V. *Handbook of developmental activities.* LaPorte, TX: Perception Developmental Research Associates, 1971.

Bluma, S., Shearer, M., Frohman, A., and Hilliard, J. *A parent's guide to early education.* Portage, WI: Cooperative Educational Service Agency, 1976.

Braley, W.T., Konicki, G., and Leedy, C.A. *Daily sensorimotor training activities.* New York: Educational Activities, 1968.

Brigance, A.H. *Diagnostic inventory of early development.* North Billerica, MA: Curriculum Associates, 1985.

Brigance, A.H. *Readiness: Strategies and practice.* North Billerica, MA: Curriculum Associates, 1985.

Cole, K. and Dale, P. . Direct language instruction and interactive language instruction with language delayed preschool children: A comparison study. *Journal of Speech and Hearing Research,* 1986, *28,* 205-217.

Coughran, L. and Goff, M. *The learning staircase assessment inventory system.* Austin, TX: Learning Concepts, 1976.

Engleman, S. and Carmine, D. *Theory of instruction: Principles and applications.* New York: Irvington, 1982.

Findlay, J., Miller, P., Pegram, A., Sanford, A., and Semrau, B. *A planning guide to the preschool curriculum.* Winston-Salem, NC: Kaplan, 1976.

Guralnick, M.J.A. and Bennett, F.C. (eds.) *The effectiveness of early intervention for at-risk and handicapped children.* New York: Academic Press, 1987.

Hart, B. and Rogers-Warren, A. Milieu approach to teaching language. In R.K. Schiefelbusch (ed.). *Language intervention strategies.* Baltimore: University Park Press, 1978.

Hui, B.M. *My little kitten (poem).* Columbia, SC: University of South Carolina, 1985.

Hui, B.M. *They wouldn't come out (poem).* Columbia, SC: University of South Carolina, 1985.

Hui, B.M. *What can it be? (poem).* Columbia, SC: University of South Carolina, 1985.

Karnes, M.B. *Helping young children develop language skills: A book of activities.* Arlington, VA: Council for Exceptional Children, 1968.

Lau, A. and Raymond, G. *Developmental assessment and instruction for success in the early years.* Columbia, SC: Daisey Associates, 1993.

Lillie, D.L. and Strum, T.M. *Carolina early learning activities: Book one.* New York: Walker and Company, 1987.

Lillie, D.L. and Strum, T.M. *Carolina early learning activities: Book two.* New York: Walker and Company, 1987.

Mann, L. *The expressive and receptive language individualization program (vol. 1).* Atlanta: Humanics, 1982.

Marzollo, J. and Lloyd, J. *Learning through play.* New York: Harper and Row, 1972.

Mattes, Larry J. (ed.) *Basic concept boosters.* Oceanside, CA: Academic Communication Associates, 1990.

McCormick, L. and Schiefelbusch, R.K. *Early language intervention.* Columbus, OH: Charles E. Merrill, 1984.

Prillaman, D. and Abbott, J.C. *Educational diagnosis and prescriptive teaching.* Belmont, CA: Pittman Learning, 1983.

Simonsson, R.J. *Psychological and developmental assessment of special children.* Boston: Allyn and Bacon, 1986.

Valencia, S., Pearson, P., Peters, C., and Wilson, K. Theory and practice in statewide reading assessment: Closing the gap. *Educational Leadership,* 1989, *46,* 57-63.

Casey, Jean. *Santa Clara plus readiness recipes: Activities kit.* Huntington Beach, CA: Richard L. Zweig Associates, 1976.

Skills Check Chart

Name	Grade/Teacher	School

		Check Date	Check Date
LANGUAGE SKILL - *VOCABULARY*			
Level A	Touches body part when given function	________	________
Level B	Names body part when given function	________	________
Level C	Expresses function of familiar object	________	________
Level D	Identifies objects belonging to categories	________	________
Level E	Names category when shown object	________	________
LANGUAGE SKILL - *CONCEPTS*			
Level A	Follows directional and positional directions	________	________
Level B	Recognizes opposites	________	________
Level C	Names colors	________	________
Level D	Names quantitative concepts	________	________
Level E	Names opposites	________	________
LANGUAGE SKILL - *SENTENCES*			
Level A	Uses sentence pattern with noun-verb-noun and prepositional phrase	________	________
Level B	Uses sentence pattern with negative	________	________
Level C	Uses sentence pattern with past tense and/or function word	________	________
Level D	Uses complete sentence to answer question	________	________
Level E	Uses sentence pattern with future tense	________	________
LANGUAGE SKILL - *STORIES*			
Level A	Tells a story about a picture	________	________
Level B	Tells a story about pictures in sequence	________	________
Level C	Responds to "Wh-" questions	________	________
Level D	Retells story after oral presentation	________	________
Level E	Places objects in sequence and explains	________	________
LANGUAGE SKILL - *LISTENING*			
Level A	Follows two-part directions	________	________
Level B	Recalls the main idea of a simple story	________	________
Level C	Follows a three-part direction in sequence	________	________
Level D	Recalls three facts from story read aloud	________	________
Level E	Identifies rhyming words	________	________

SCORING

+ = Performs task   0 = Fails to perform task

Language Scope and Sequence

INSTRUCTION AGE	ACTIVITY LEVEL	VOCABULARY	CONCEPTS	SENTENCES	STORIES	LISTENING
3.0	A	Touches body part when given function	Follows directional and positional words	Uses sentence patterns with N-V-N+ prepositional phrase	Tells story about a picture	Follows two-part directions
3.5	B	Names body part when given function	Recognizes opposites	Uses sentence patterns with a negative	Tells story about pictures in sequence	Recalls the main idea of a story
4.0	C	Expresses function of selected objects	Names colors	Uses sentence patterns with past tense / function word	Responds to "wh-" questions	Follows a three-part direction in sequence
4.5	D	Identifies objects in categories	Names quantitative concepts	Uses complete sentences to answer questions	Retells story after oral presentation	Recalls three facts from a story
5.0	E	Names category of objects	Names opposites	Uses sentence patterns with future tense	Sequences objects and tells how done	Identifies rhyming words

LILAC

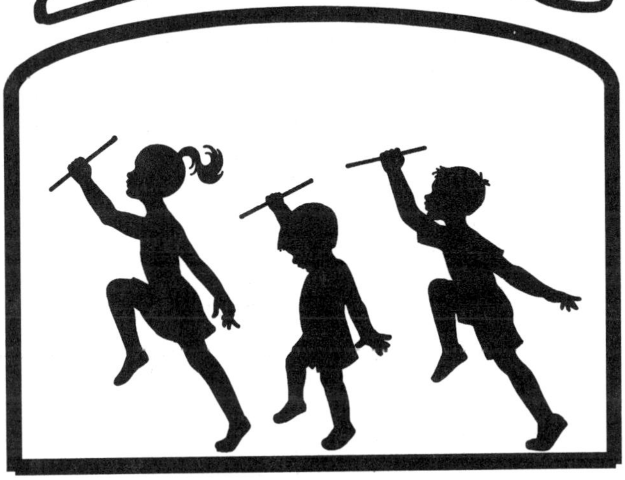

Levels A - E

Primary: Level A

Activity 1: Body Parts

Objective: To touch corresponding body parts (such as eyes, ears, mouth, nose, feet, legs, hands, and fingers) when given function

Materials: Doll or stuffed toy with eyes, nose, and mouth

EYES and EARS

1. These are my eyes. Point to your eyes. I will touch the doll's eyes. Now you touch the doll's eyes.

   Eyes are the body part we see with. Put your hands over your eyes. Can you see? Point to the body part you see with. Do you see with your eyes? Do you see with your ears? Do you see with your mouth? Do you see with your nose? Again, let's point to the body part you see with.

   Now, let's sing a song (tune of "Mulberry Bush"):

   This is the way I point to my eyes, point to my eyes, point to my eyes.
   This is the way I point to my eyes, early in the morning.
   Blink, blink, blink your eyes.
   Blink your eyes, blink your eyes.
   Blink, blink, blink your eyes,
   Blink your eyes together.

2. These are my ears. Point to your ears. I will touch the doll's ears. Now you touch the doll's ears. You use your ears to hear things with. Listen.

   Knock on the table. What did you hear? Did you hear me knock? You used your ears to hear with. Now, put your hands over your ears.

   Knock softly on the table. Did you hear me knock? You could not because you had your ears covered, and your ears are what you hear with. Point to the part of your body you hear with. Do not let me trick you. Listen. Do you hear with your ears? Do you hear with your eyes? Do you hear with your mouth?

   Make more familiar sounds, such as snapping fingers, stamping feet, clapping hands, humming, knocking, and tapping pencil. What did you hear? Point to the body part you hear with. Now listen carefully.

   Make a familiar animal sound, such as baa, moo, quack, arf, or meow. What animal makes that sound? Touch the body part that you hear with.

NOSE

Materials: Items that smell (such as soap, lotion, onion, pepper, flower, orange slice) *(CAUTION: Verify that children have no allergies being doing this activity.)*

3. This is my nose. Point to your nose. I will touch the doll's nose. Now you touch the doll's nose. You use your nose to smell things with.

Display items that smell.

You used your nose to smell with. What did you smell?

Allow children to smell the object, identify the body part they smell with, and name each object.

Point to the part of your body you smell with. Do not let me trick you. Listen. Do you smell with your ears? Do you smell with your nose? Do you smell with your mouth?

MOUTH

4. This is my mouth. Point to your mouth. I will touch the doll's mouth. Now you touch the doll's mouth. You use your mouth to taste and eat with as well as talk with.

What is your favorite food?

What part of your body do you eat with? What part of your body do you talk with? Point to the part of your body you eat with. Do not let me trick you. Listen. Do you eat with your nose? Do you eat with your eyes? Do you eat with your mouth?

I am going to tell you a story. Listen, because I am going to ask you what the boy does with his mouth in the story.

A little boy goes to visit his grandmother. On the way he whistles a happy tune. When he gets to his grandmother's, he kisses his grandmother hello. She gives him cookies to eat. They laugh and talk all day. Then, he kisses her goodbye and goes home.

Tell me what the little boy did with his mouth.

FACE

Materials: Paper with large circle drawn on it
Cut-out eyes, ears, nose, and mouth
Glue

5. Let's quickly review:

   What body part do we see with?
   What body part do we hear with?
   What body part do we smell with?
   What body part do we talk or eat with?

   Now we each are going to make a face with the body parts we know. I am going to put my face together. Watch me carefully.

   This is my mouth. We eat and talk with our mouths.
   This is my nose. We smell with our noses.
   These are my ears. We hear with our ears.
   And these are my eyes. We see with our eyes.

   I want you to make a face just like mine. *Make faces.* Now that our faces are complete, let's point to each part and talk about what it does. Then, let's sing a song (tune of "If You're Happy and You Know It"):

   If you're happy and you know it, touch your eyes.
   If you're happy and you know it, touch your eyes.
   If you're happy and you know it, then your face will surely show it.
   If you're happy and you know it, touch your eyes.
   Continue verses with ears, nose, and mouth.

HANDS

6. These are my hands. Show me your hands. Let's play a game. Do what I do. We can do all these things with our hands.

   Clap your hands.
   Raise one hand.
   Wave two hands.
   Raise two hands.
   Wave one hand.
   Shake one hand.
   Wiggle two hands.
   Shake two hands.
   Wiggle one hand.

   After the group follows the directions with their hands, ask children to follow the directions by themselves, one at a time.

Parts of a Face

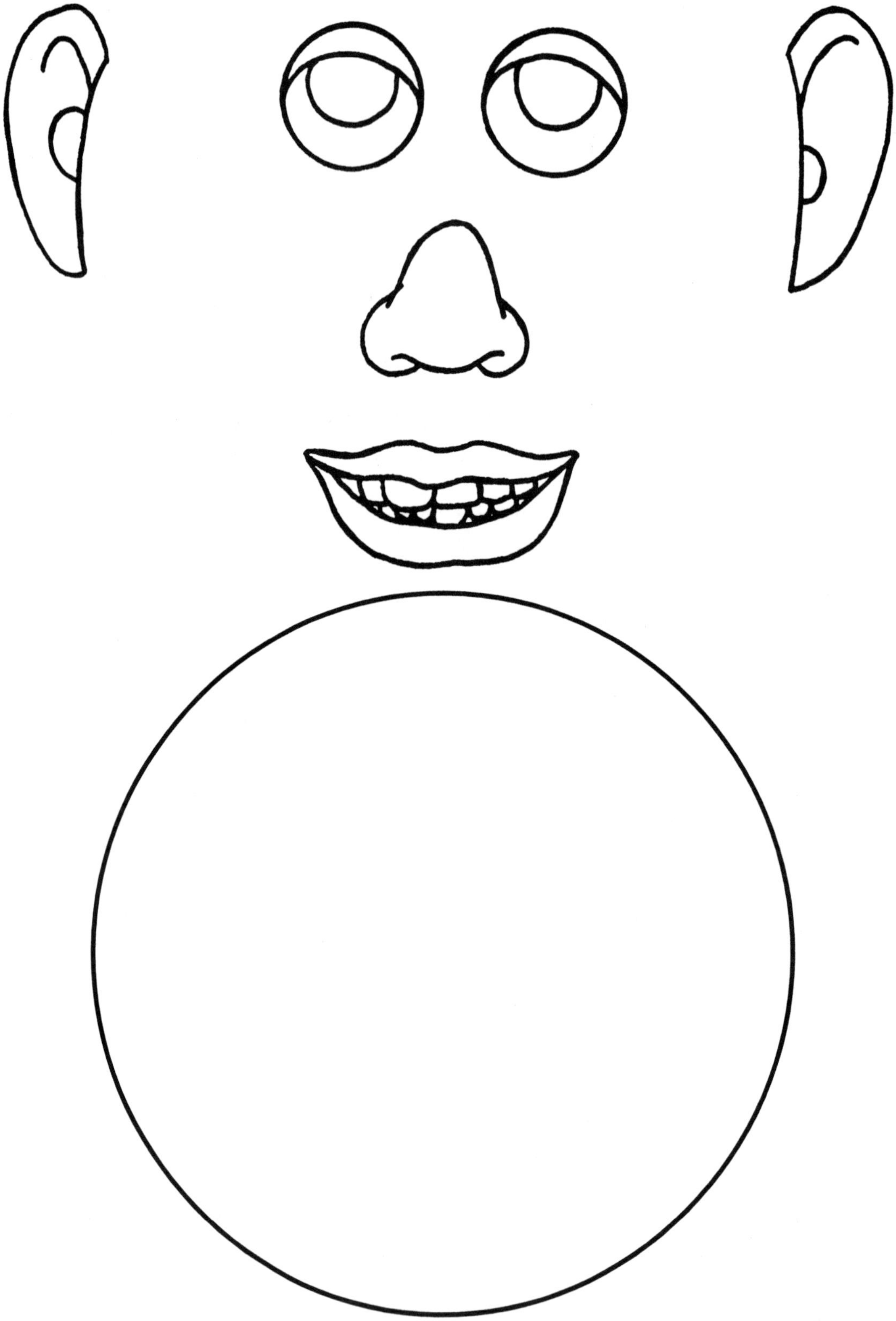

Let's do a finger-play exercise now:

Open them, shut them.
Open them, shut them.
Give a little clap.
Open them, shut them.
Open them, shut them.
Put them in your lap.
Creep them, creep them
Up to your mouth –
Do not let your fingers in.

FINGERS and ARMS

7. These are my fingers. Let's point to our fingers. Now, point to your neighbor's fingers. You are pointing with your fingers. Specifically, we point with our pointer finger.

This is your pointer finger.
This is your thumb.
This is your little finger.
Those are the parts of your hands.
Let's wiggle your fingers.
Let's walk our fingers on the table like spiders.
Where are your fingers?
Where is your pointer finger?
Where is your little finger?
Where is your thumb?

8. Here are my arms. Where are your arms? Let's raise our arms up high. Point to your neighbor's arms. We can raise our arms in the air. We can shake, swing, and fold our arms and put them behind our backs. Now let's do activities with our arms. Listen and do these:

Swing your arms.
Raise them in the air.
Fold them in front of you.
Put them behind your back.
Now, put them on your knees.

Now, let's sing a song (tune of "Mulberry Bush"):

This is the way I swing my arms, swing my arms, swing my arms.
This is the way I swing my arms, early in the morning.
Swing, swing, swing, my arms. Swing my arms, swing my arms,
Swing, swing, swing my arms, early in the morning.
Continue with fold my arms, wave my arms, and shake my arms.

LEGS and FEET

Materials: Chair

9. These are my feet. We use feet to walk, to run, to kick, and to put on shoes. These are my legs. We use legs to walk, to run, to jump, and to bend up and down.

    Everyone, touch your legs. Now, touch your feet. Watch what I do. I will stand behind the chair. I will walk around the chair. I will put my foot on the chair. Now, listen to what I say, and do exactly what I say to do with your legs and feet.

    Point to the part(s) of your body that you run with.
    Point to the part(s) of your body that you walk with.
    Point to the part(s) of your body that you kick with.
    Point to the part(s) of your body that you put shoes on.
    Point to the part(s) of your body that you jump with.
    Point to the part(s) of your body that you bend.

    Let's run. I am running in place with my feet. You do it too.
    What are we doing with our feet?

    Continue with activities to do with legs and feet, such as walk, run, skip, hop, jump, and tiptoe.

BODY

Materials: Crayons or felt-tip markers
Outline of child's body drawn on paper (including head, trunk, arms, hands, legs, and feet)

10. *Review all the body parts introduced in previous activities. Ask each child to respond to directions by touching the appropriate body parts.*

    Touch the part(s) of your body that you see with.
    Touch the part(s) of your body that you hear with.
    Touch the part(s) of your body that you talk or eat with.
    Touch the part(s) of your body that you smell with.
    Touch the part(s) of your body that you run with.
    Touch the part(s) of your body that you clap with.
    Touch the part(s) of your body that you point with.
    Touch the part(s) of your body that you kick a ball with.

    Now, let's color the body parts on this picture as we talk about them. *Distribute outlines and crayons. Ask children to color body parts as they discuss each part's use.*

Body

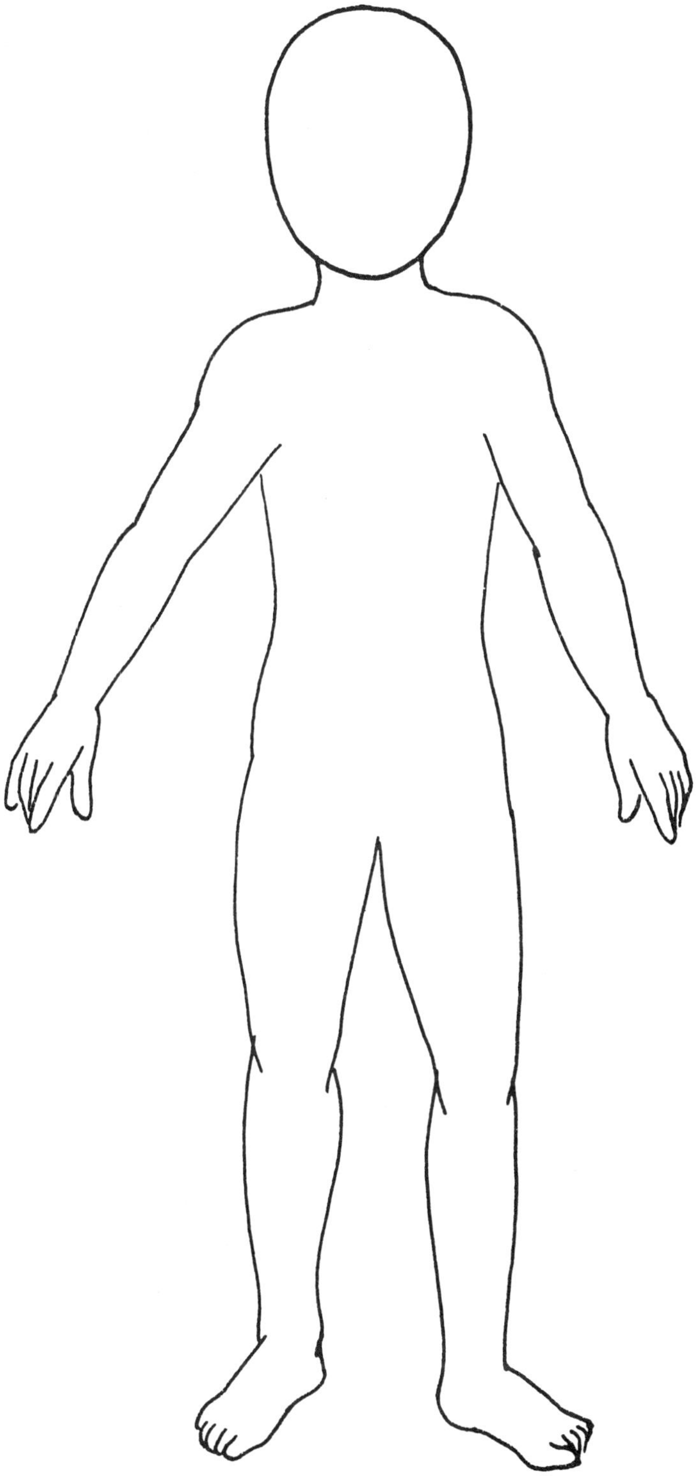

Let's learn and do a chant. Listen.

Who feels happy?
Who feels gay?
All who do, clap your hands this way.

Continue with other verses:

Wiggle your fingers.
Stamp your feet.
Swing your arms.
Touch your legs.
Blink your eyes.
Touch your nose.
Open your mouth.
Touch your ears.

If time allows, make outlines of each child's body on butcher paper and label them. (You may also use flannel board body and parts.) Encourage the children to take turns placing the body parts appropriately and discussing their actions as they do them.

PROGRESS CHECK

Materials: None

Observe the children as they follow these directions:

Touch the part(s) of your body that you kick a ball with.
Touch the part(s) of your body that you run with.
Touch the part(s) of your body that you see with.
Touch the part(s) of your body that you hear with.
Touch the part(s) of your body that you smell with.
Touch the part(s) of your body that you clap with.
Touch the part(s) of your body that you eat or talk with.
Touch the part(s) of your body that you raise in the air.
Touch the part(s) of your body that you point with.

Scoring:

+	Identifies all nine body parts correctly
0	Fails to identify all nine body parts correctly

Primary: Level A

Activity 2: Directional and Positional Concepts

Objective: To follow directions containing directional/positional words, such as "out," "on," "up," "down," "under," "top," "middle," "bottom," and "in"

Materials: Newspaper
Masking tape

UP and DOWN

1. *Hold up a ball made of crumpled newspaper and masking tape.*

   I have a ball. I made the ball from newspaper and masking tape. Now, we will each make our own ball out of newspaper and tape.

   Distribute newspaper already crumpled into a ball and help each child place masking tape around the ball.

   Look, I am holding my ball *up* high.
   Now, I am holding my ball *down* low.
   Everyone look.
   Where am I holding my ball?
   Where am I holding my ball now?

   Emphasize to the children the importance of using complete sentences when answering questions. ("You are holding your ball up high." "I am holding my ball up high.")

2. We can do the same *up* and *down* directions with our balls. Watch. I am putting my ball *up* on the shelf. Say with me: "You are putting your ball *up* on the shelf." Now, I am putting my ball *down* off the shelf. Say with me: "You are putting your ball *down* off the shelf." Follow these directions. Listen.

   ____________________ *(child's name),* please put your ball *on* the shelf.

   Everyone. Where is ____________________'s ball?

   Now, ____________________, take your ball *down* off the shelf.

   Where is ____________________'s ball now?

   Allow children to put their balls up on and down off the shelf. Then, give them directions, such as hold hands up and down, hold one hand up and down, and hold a foot up and down.

Materials: Large cardboard box
Paper balls
Small cardboard box

3. *Seat the children on the floor in a circle. Show the children the big box. Get in the box. Say:* I am in the box. Where am I?

   Get out of the box. I am now out of the box. Where am I?

   Let's everyone try.

   Let each of the children take a turn getting into and out of the big box. The children must respond each time to the question asking where they are.

   > Now, let's get the little box. I am going to put the ball in the box, but this ball is out of the box.

   Allow the children to put a ball in different places. Ask them to tell where the ball is located in relation to the box each time the ball is moved.

ON, BESIDE, and UNDER

Materials:		
	Table	Chair
	Ball	Box
	Book	Block

4. *Using a table and an object, demonstrate placement of the object "on" the table, "under" the table, and "beside" the table, saying:*

   > This block in *on* the table.
   > This box is *under* the chair.
   > This chair is *beside* the table.

   Ask children individually to demonstrate each of these. Now, let's take turns being leader.

   Let each child tell the other children what to do with specific objects. Help the leader make sure they use the "on," "beside," and "under" words.

Materials: Ball made of newspaper
Box
Construction paper eyes and whiskers for a cat
Glue

5. Watch me while I make my ball into a cat.

Put "eyes" and "whiskers" on the ball, then use the cat and the box to tell the following story. While telling the story, perform appropriate movements, using gestures demonstrating the concepts, such as "out," "beside," "up," "on," "down," "under," and "in:"

> One day two children went to school. Their cat was lonely inside so he went out and sat beside the house. A dog came along and frightened their cat. So, the cat ran up and sat on the roof. The cat watched until the dog left, and then he came down. Soon, the cat heard noises that sounded like mice under the house. So, he went under the house to look for mice. The cat searched but could not find the mice, so he sat beside the house to rest. Soon the two children came home from school. They all went in the house for cookies and milk *(B.M. Hui).*

Now, let's all do what I did while I read the story again for you. You try.

Allow children, either individually or as a group, to perform the appropriate actions while you read the story aloud.

TOP, MIDDLE, and BOTTOM

Materials: Step stool
Classroom shelves with toys on top, middle, and bottom shelves

6. *Using a step stool, demonstrate:*

I am sitting on the *top* step. Now, I am sitting on the *bottom* step. I am sitting on the *middle* step now. Let's let you try. Listen.

Give each child individual directions to sit on the "top," "middle," and "bottom" steps. Demonstrate, using the shelves with toys.

This doll is on the *top* shelf. This doll is on the *middle* shelf, and this doll in on the *bottom* shelf.

Your turn. You be the leader and put a toy on a shelf. When you are done, we will tell you where the toy is.

Let each child place the doll appropriately while other children tell where it is.

I have a game. Please follow my directions. Ready? *Give directions:*

Put your hands on *top* of your head.
Put your hands on the *bottom* of your feet.
Put your hands on the *middle* of your body.
Continue by varying statements.

Materials: Flannel board
Two each of several cut-outs, such as apples, bananas, stars, balls, or hearts

7. I am putting this apple at the *top* of the board. I will put this star in the *middle* of the board. I will put this ball at the *bottom* of the board.

Where did I put the star?
Where did I put the apple?
Where did I put the ball?

Let each child answer questions independently. Praise. Give each child a cut-out.

Put your cut-out on the board in a certain place. Then, one of us will tell you where you put your shape.

Allow each child to put one shape on the board and tell where it was placed.

Now, you be the leader and tell us where to put our objects on the board.

Materials: Flannel board
Cut-out shapes of familiar objects
Yarn

8. *Place yarn in the shape of a circle on the flannel board. Place each cut-out on the board.*

I will put the apple *in* the circle.
I am going to put the star *beside* the circle.
I am putting the ball *under* the circle.
Now, I am going to put the banana on *top* of the circle.

Ask each child:

Where is the apple?
Where is the banana?
Where is the ball?
Where is the star?

Think of a place for an object to go *on* the board, and then tell us where it is.

Objects: Apple, Star, Heart, Ball, Umbrella, Banana

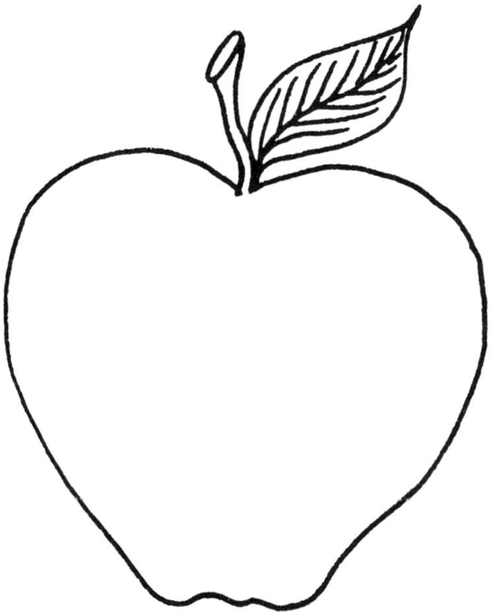

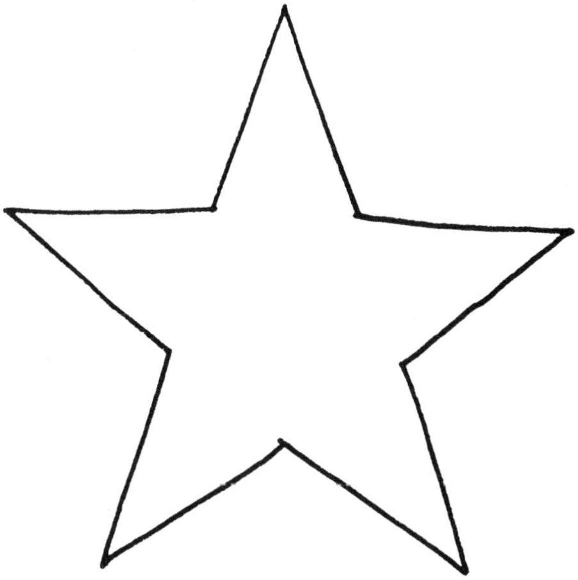

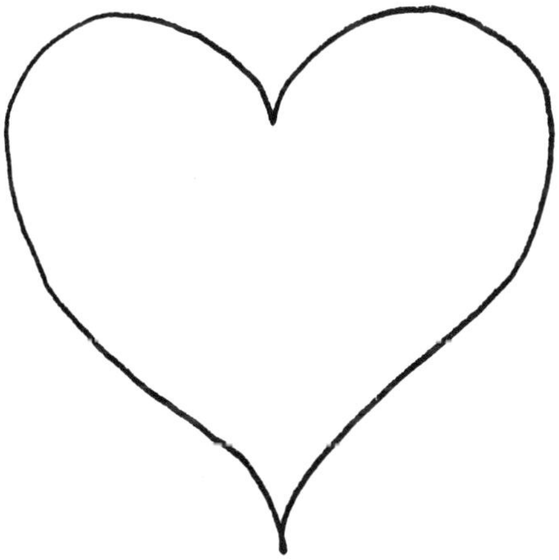

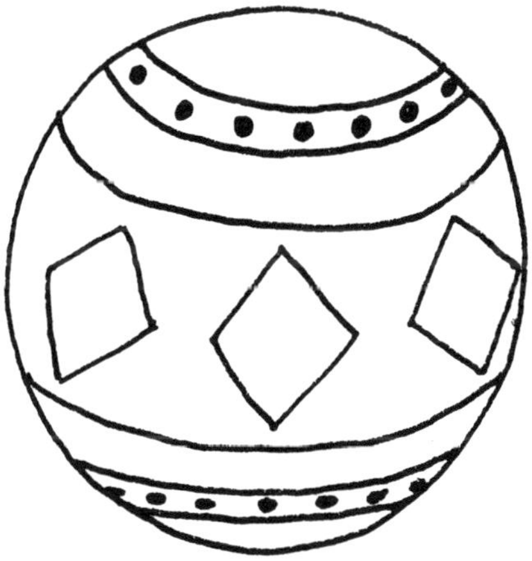

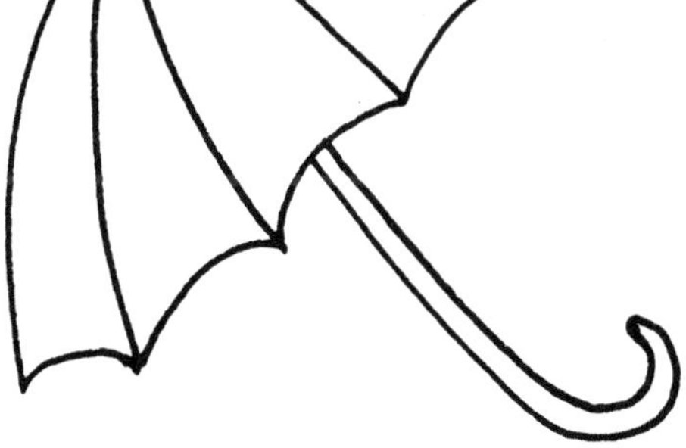

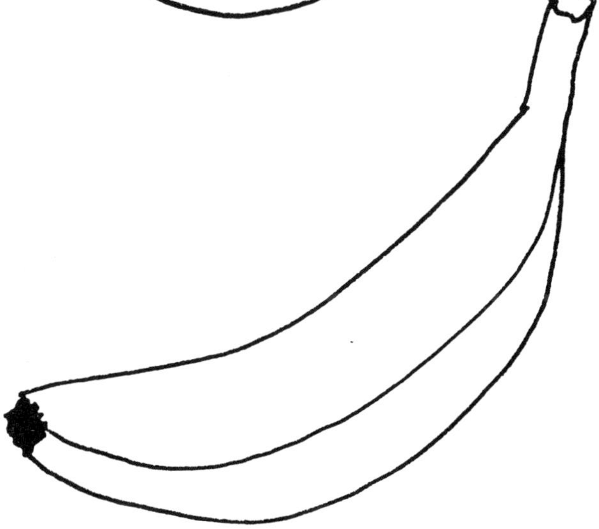

DIRECTIONAL / POSITIONAL CONCEPTS

Materials: Flannel board and cut-outs of a cat, house, and tree

9. I have a story to tell you. Listen. *Place cat appropriately on flannel board during story.*

   One day two children went to school. Their cat went outside and sat beside the house. A dog came along and frightened the cat. The cat ran up the side of the house and sat on the roof. He watched until the dog left, and then came down. Soon he heard noises under the house that sounded like mice. So, the cat went under the house to look for them. He searched but could not find them. So he went back outside and sat beside the house to rest. Then he heard the dog coming back, so he ran to the top of a tree. The cat waited until he felt a little safer, then he went down to the middle of the tree. A little later he went down to the bottom of the tree. Soon, the two children came home from school, and they all went in the house for a snack *(B.M. Hui).*

   Ask children questions about where the cat was located at different times. Let each child answer. I will tell the story again, but this time you take turns moving the cat on the board.

10. Let's sing a song (tune of "This Is the Way We Wash Our Clothes"):

    My little fingers are on the table,
    On the table, on the table.
    My little fingers are on the table.
    Now they are in my lap.
    (Repeat with other verses, such as under the table, up so high, down low, and on top of my head.)

PROGRESS CHECK

Materials: Flannel board and cut-out shapes of familiar objects

Observe the children performing the following:

Put the ball at the *top* of the board.
Put the star in the *middle* of the board.
Now, put the heart *beside* the star.
Put the apple at the *bottom* of the board.
Put the umbrella *under* the ball.
Put the banana *over* the apple.

Scoring:

+	Follows all directions correctly
0	Fails to follow all directions correctly

Story: Cat, Dog, House, and Tree

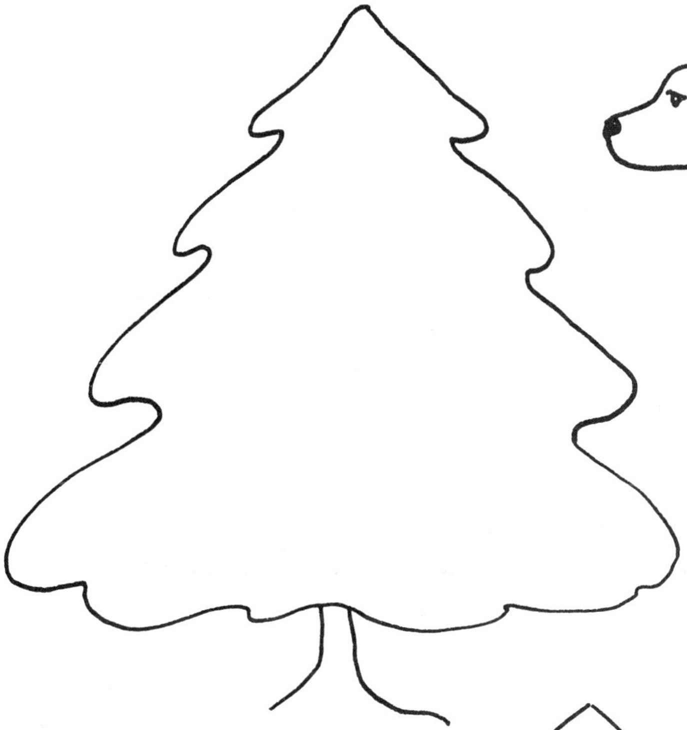

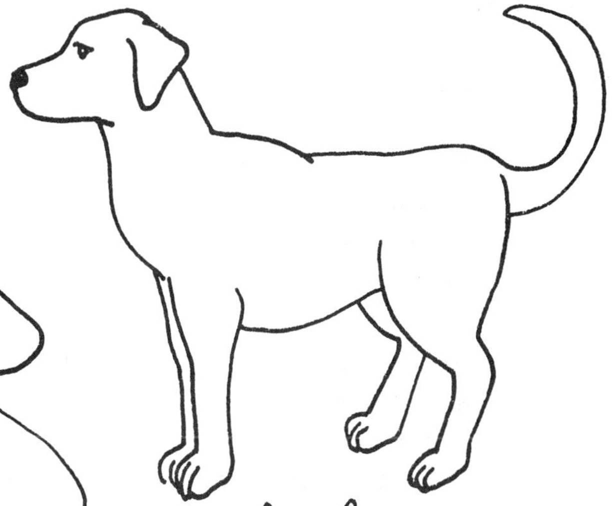

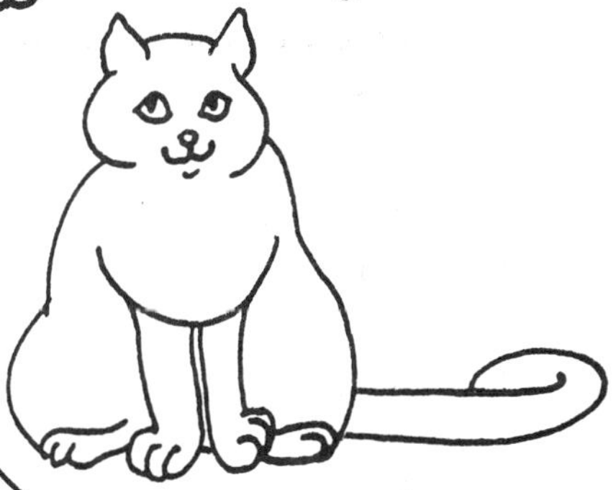

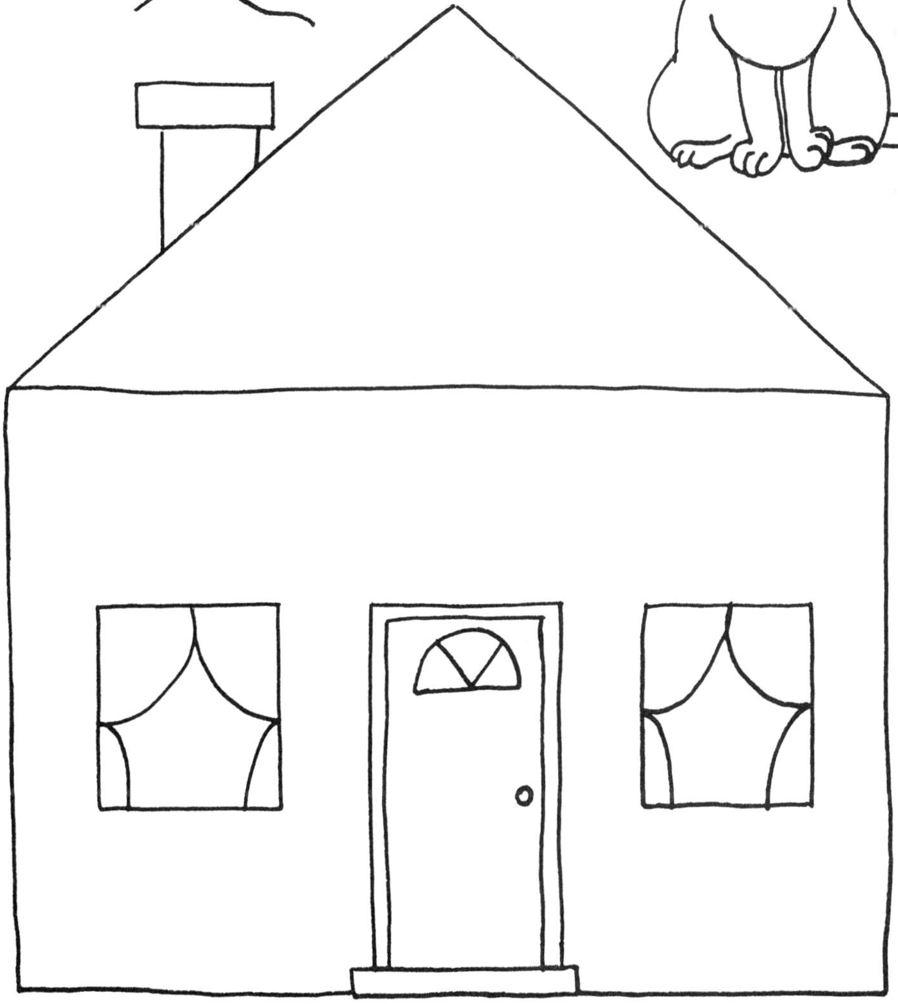

Primary: Level A

Activity 3: Sentences

Objective: To use sentence patterns with noun-verb-noun and prepositional phrase

Materials: Grocery bag; Pictures of food; Empty boxes and cans with labels; Book of nursery rhymes

1. Listen, my name is Ms./Mr. ____________________. If you ask me my name, I will say, "My name is Ms./Mr. ____________________." Now, you tell me your name when I ask, "What is your name?" *Ask children their names. Make sure they answer in a complete sentence.*

2. *Use a grocery bag filled with items, such as empty cereal boxes, soup cans, and vegetable cans.*

   We are going to pretend we are going grocery shopping. I am going to buy some cereal. *Take a cereal box out of bag.* Now, you reach into the bag and tell me what you are going to buy. Remember to use complete sentences.

   Let each child take a turn in choosing something from the bag and responding in complete sentences, such as "I am going to buy a can of peaches."

3. Let's say a nursery rhyme together. *Select any nursery rhyme and say it together. (Remember to emphasize complete sentences.)*

Materials: Grocery bag; Toys (or pictures of toys)

4. I like to eat pizza *(personalize).* Let's talk about what you like to eat. *Ask:* What do you like to eat? Remember to use complete sentences. (*Encourage each child to respond using a complete sentence.*)

5. Now let's go on a shopping trip like we did earlier. But this time, let's go to the toy store. *Place the toys or pictures of toys in a bag.*

   > Choose something from the bag to "buy" at the store. Then, tell me what you bought. Remember to use complete sentences.

   Allow each child to reach in the bag and respond to the question.

   Let's say another rhyme. *Choose another rhyme; emphasize speaking in complete sentences.*

Foods

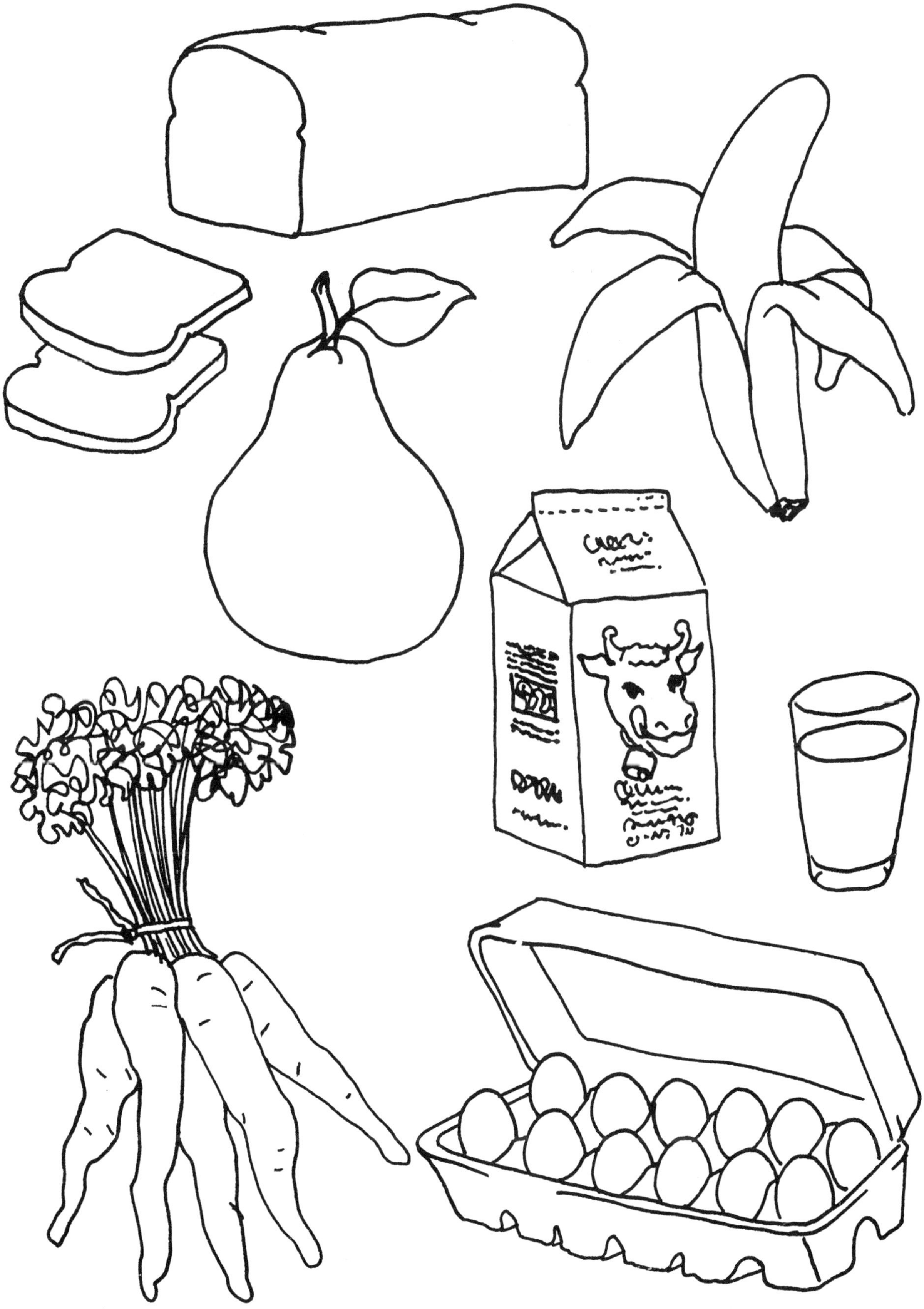

Toys

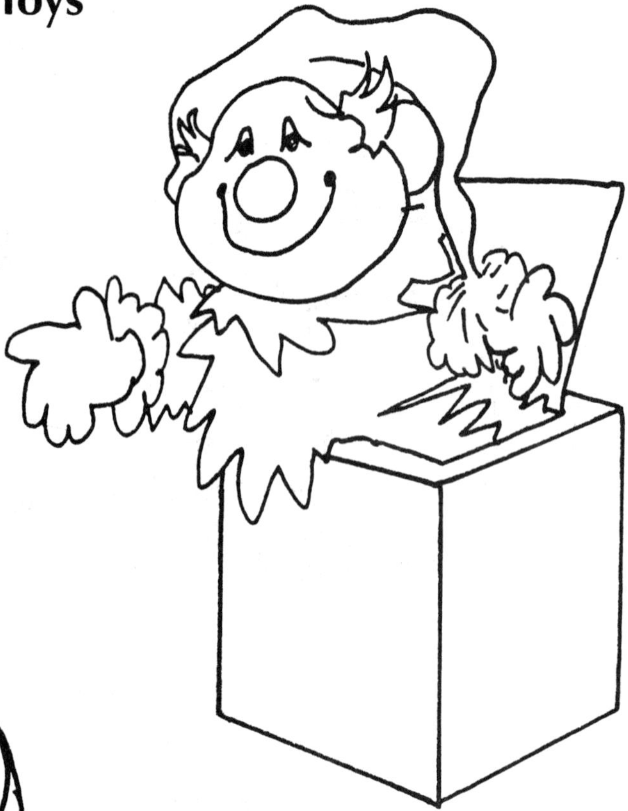

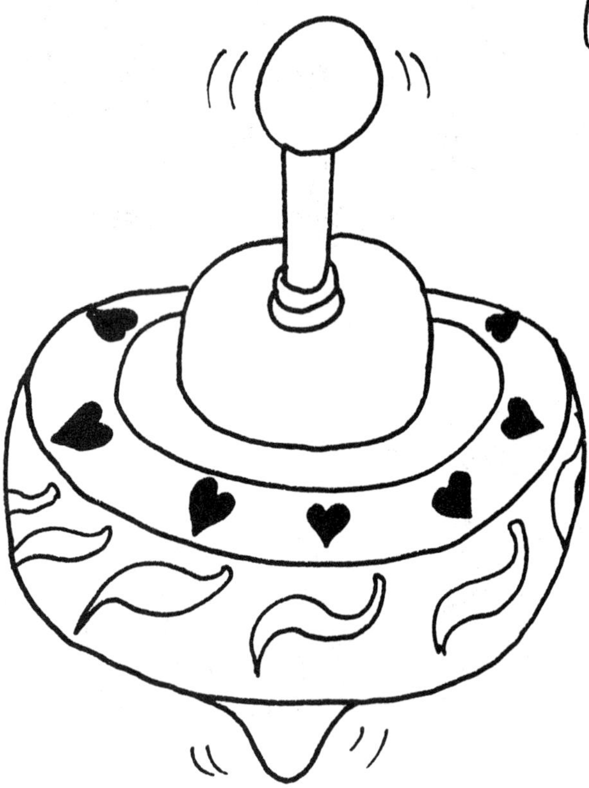

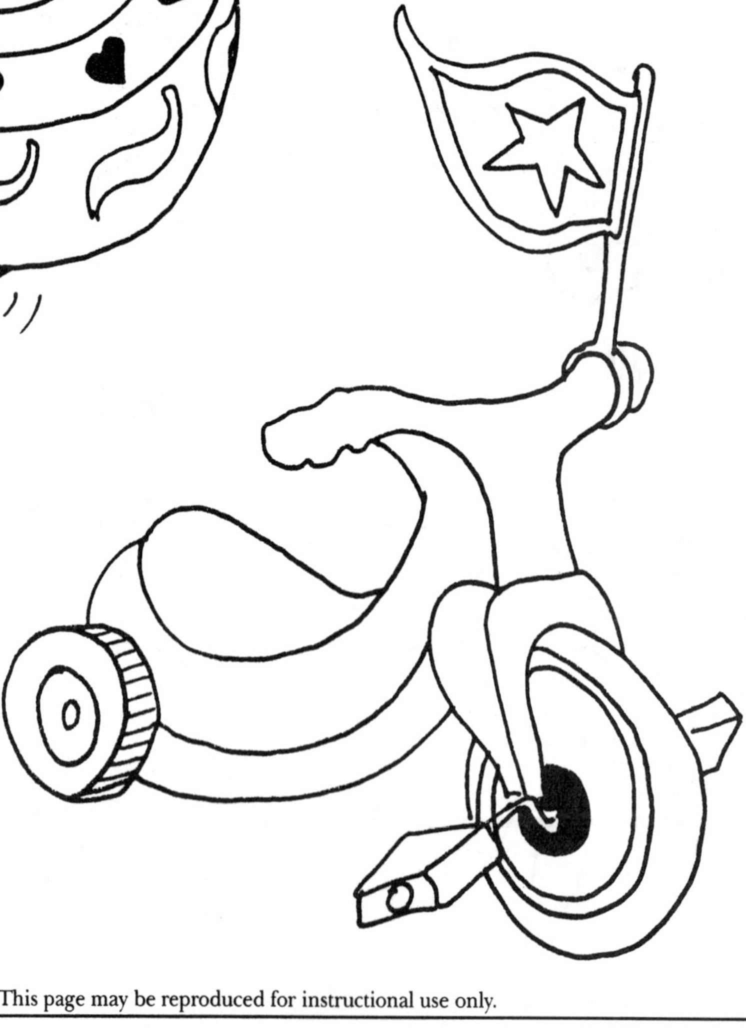

Animals

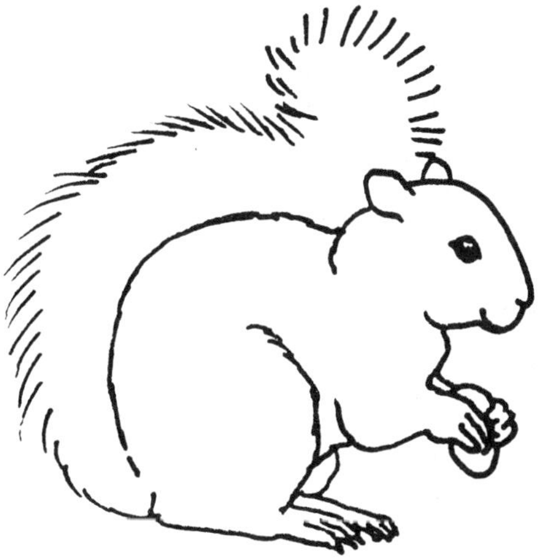

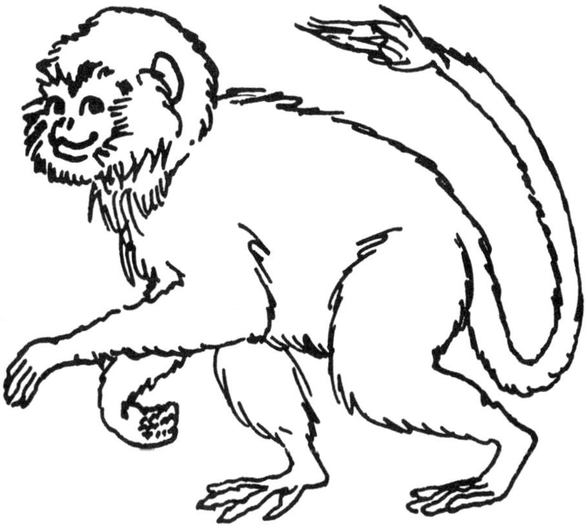

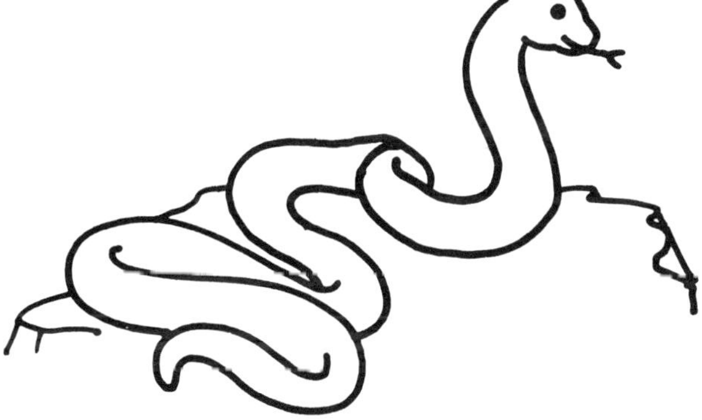

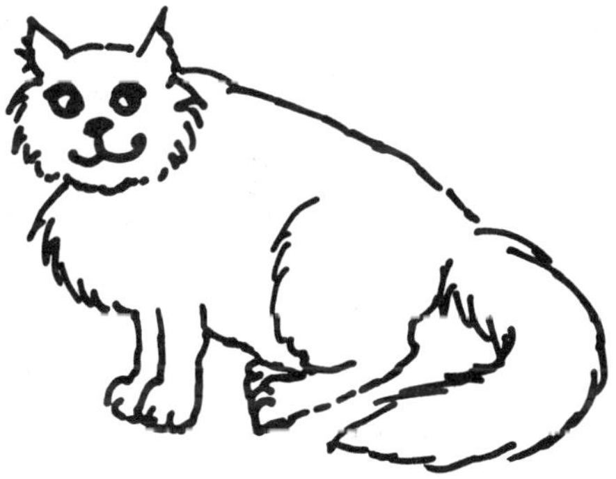

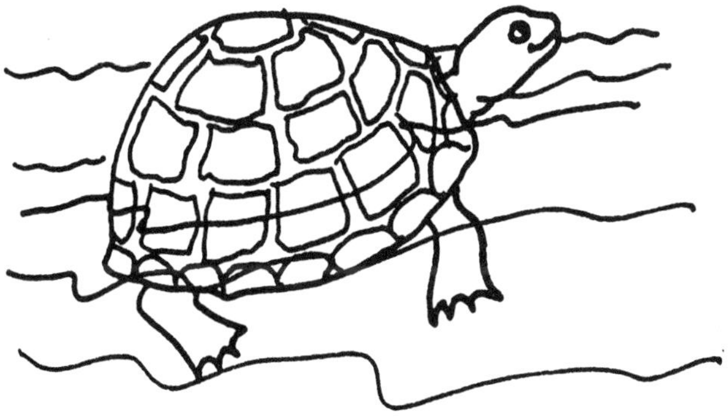

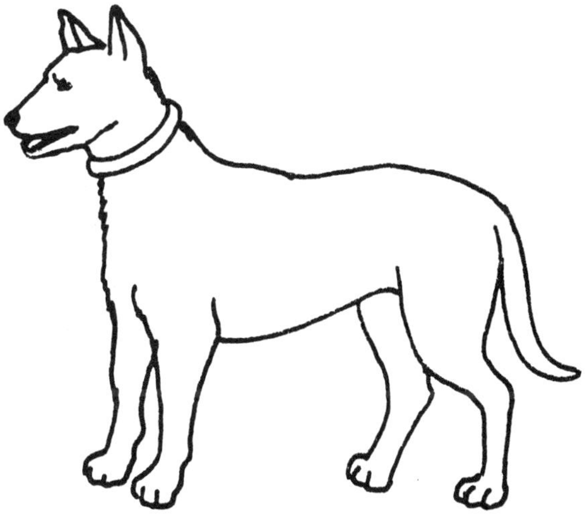

Materials: Two puppets
Doll or teddy bear
Doll furniture
Large wagon or truck
Tape recorder

6. I have a puppet. I can talk to my puppet, and it can talk to me. *Demonstrate the puppet responding in complete sentences.*

   "What is your name?" "My name is ____________________." Now, you try talking to the puppet.

   Allow the children to talk to the puppet – both asking and receiving questions.

   Now, let's see what we can do to help our doll.
   She is very tired. Let's put her to bed.
   The doll could say, "I am sleeping in the bed."

   Continue to use other toys, such as the bear and the wagon, to emphasize complete sentences. Ask each child to answer questions about what the toy is doing, such as, "The bear is riding in the wagon." What does the bear say, "I am riding in the wagon."

   While the children are talking, use the tape recorder to record their sentences, then let them listen to the sentences recorded.

Materials: Grocery bag
Toy animals (or pictures of animals)

7. Now, let's go on a "Shopping Trip."

   I have stuffed animals (or pictures of animals) in my bag. We are going to the pet store to buy animals. *Reach in the bag and take out a picture or toy.* I am going to buy a dog *(personalize according to the picture pulled out).* See how I used a complete sentence to say what I am going to buy. Now, you try.

   Allow each child the opportunity to play.

   Let's work on a new nursery rhyme.

   Select a new rhyme, and repeat it as a group. Emphasize the use of complete sentences. Repeat all previously learned rhymes.

Materials: Flannel board
Cut-outs of common objects, such as ball, box, or other objects

8. *Place cut-outs on the flannel board in different positions.*

The ball is in the corner of the board. Where is the ball?
The ball is at the bottom. Where is the ball?
The ball is in the middle. Where is the ball?
Now, you tell me where the ball is as I move it around.

Allow each child to give responses independently.

Materials: Masking tape

9. *Give the children a small piece of masking tape. Say*: Put your piece of tape somewhere on your body where everyone can see the tape. I will put my piece of tape on my nose. *Say:* My tape is on my nose. Where is your tape? *Ask each child individually to respond in complete sentences.*

10. I am wearing a sweater *(personalize all sentences). Point to a particular child. Say:* You are wearing blue socks. *Turn to the child next to you and talk about what that child is wearing. Say:* I am going to ask one of you to tell me something that ______________ is wearing. Remember to say what the child is wearing in a complete sentence. *Give each child an opportunity to tell something that one of their neighbors is wearing.*

PROGRESS CHECK

Materials: Flannel board
Cut-outs of common objects

Select one of the cut-outs. Say (for example): I have a ball. My ball is in the middle of the board. *Place the ball in the middle of the board.*

Select a cut-out and put it on the board. Say: Now, tell me where it is. Remember to use a complete sentence. *Ask the child to place and tell where three objects are located.*

Scoring:

+	Responds in complete sentences three times
0	Fails to respond in complete sentences three times

Primary: Level A

Activity 4: Stories

Objective: To tell a story about a picture

Materials:
Large box
Tape recorder
Dry cereals to use as food
Dog bowl
Pictures of animals (page 35)

ACTIONS

1. Let's pretend I am a duck. I can walk like a duck. I say, "Quack, quack." I am hungry. *Eat or pretend to eat dry cereal in a bowl.* I go into my house. *Go into the boxes.*

   Now, pretend you are a duck, and tell us a story about yourself. *Allow each child the opportunity to pretend to be a duck and talk.*

   Repeat the creative drama with other animals, such as dog, cat, rabbit, pig, chicken, snake, elephant, cow, horse, sheep, and/or frog.

2. *Place several pictures of familiar animals on the table in front of the children.*

   I'm thinking of something soft and fuzzy; it says, "Meow." What is it? *Allow all children to guess.* That is right. It is a cat.

   Continue with riddles. Allow each child to answer individually at least two times.

   Now, you be the leader, and tell us an animal riddle to solve. *Ask the children to take turns telling riddles to the others.*

3. *Place pictures of animals face down on the table.*

   Let's tell stories about animals. Choose a picture of an animal, and tell us about the animal you chose. You can tell us its name, its color, where the animal lives, what the animal eats, or anything else about it. *Tape record the children's stories. Play stories for them when they are finished.*

4. I have a song for us. Now, let's sing a song (tune of "Mulberry Bush"):

   This is the way we wash our face,
   Wash our face, wash our face.
   This is the way we wash our face,
   Early in the morning.
   (Add other actions to make additional verses for the song.)

Materials: Pictures showing actions

5. *Show pictures to children. Describe action in each picture with a one-sentence story.*

   The boy is eating his lunch.
   This girl is swinging on the swing.

   Now, you choose a picture, and tell us one thing that is happening in the picture. *Draw a simple picture on a chalkboard or flip chart.* Tell me about this picture. Now, I want you to draw a picture, and tell us about it. *Allow each child a turn.*

Materials: Clay or similar material

6. *Give each child some clay. Say:* I am going to make something with my clay. Can you guess what I am making?

   Make an animal. Allow children to guess. Say: Yes, I made a ___________________.

   Now, you make something, and we will guess what you made. *Allow each child to form objects, and then tell about them.*

Materials: Illustrated nursery rhymc book

7. *Tell nursery rhymes while showing pictures. Encourage children to repeat rhymes with you by saying, "Say these rhymes with me."*

PROGRESS CHECK

Materials: Pictures that show actions

Place action pictures face down on the table. Say: Choose a picture, then tell me two things about it.

Scoring:

+	Tells two things about picture without prompts
0	Fails to tell two things without prompts

Action Pictures

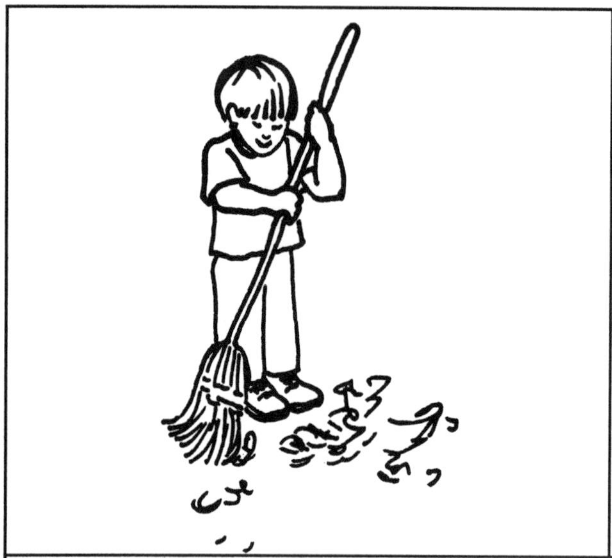
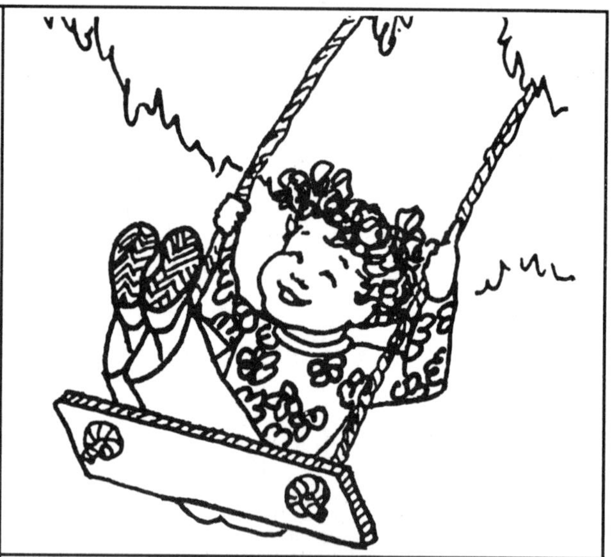
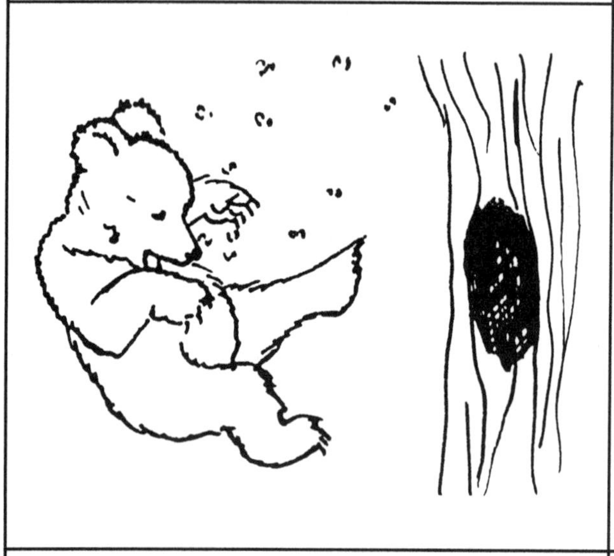
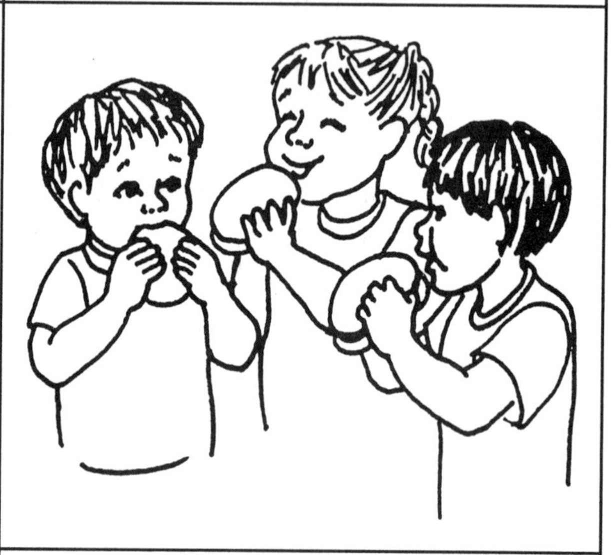
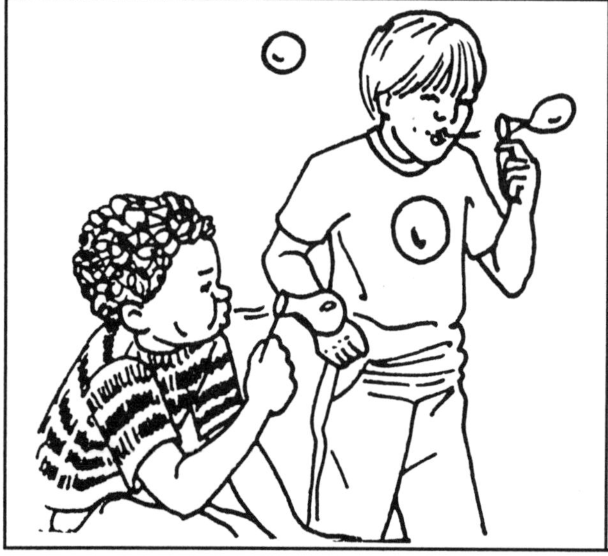
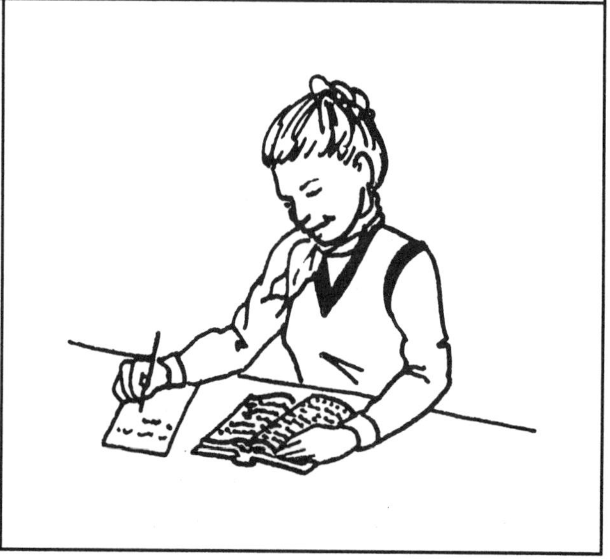

Primary: Level A

Activity 5: Following Directions

Objective: To follow two-part directions

Materials: None

1. *Group the children in a circle.*

   Today, we are going to play a game called "This Is the Way." *Demonstrate the game by doing the actions at the same time as the words.*

   This is the way I wash my hands,
   Wash my hands, wash my hands.
   This is the way I wash my hands
   Before I come to school.

   Continue with: Brush my teeth, brush my hair, put on my shirt, eat my breakfast, put on my shoes, wash my face, and get on the bus.

   Choose one child at a time to follow a direction as it is spoken. Choose a child to demonstrate an action, but do not let the rest of the group know what that child will be acting. Encourage the other children to guess the action.

2. We are going to play a game. You must listen carefully and do what I say when I call your name. Listen.

   Put your hands on your head and wiggle your fingers.
   Pat your knees, and then sit on your hands.

   Ask individual children to perform a specified action when their names are called.

   Listen. Again, do what I say when I call your name.
   Put your hands on your head and wiggle your fingers.
   Pat your knees and then sit on your hands.

   Allow each child the opportunity to complete a two-part direction. Let's see if we can follow the directions in my song. Listen, let's stand up. Are you ready? Here we go.

   Teddy bear, teddy bear, turn around.
   Teddy bear, teddy bear, touch the ground.
   Teddy bear, teddy bear, show your shoe.
   Teddy bear, teddy bear, that will do.

Materials: Plastic bowl, Cup, Blanket, Large box, Familiar toys, Spoon, Hair brush, Shirt that buttons, Paper bag

3. *Place objects on table.* We are going to play a game. I will call your name and ask you to pretend to do two things. See if you can do them. Ready? *Ask each child by name.*

    ____________________, wash your hands. Now, dry them.

    ____________________, eat your cereal. Now, drink the milk.

    ____________________, put on your shirt. Now, button your shirt.

    I am going to tell you two things to do. But this time I will tell you both directions at the same time. Listen carefully, so you can remember what to do. Ready?

    ____________________, pick up the doll and bring it to me.

    ____________________, pick up the blue car and put it in the box.

    Continue to give simple two-part directions until each child has had several turns.

4. I have a finger play to teach you. Listen, and I will show you how to do it.

    Here are Grandma's glasses *(put fingers around eyes).*
    Here is Grandma's hat *(put hands on head).*
    Here is the way she folds her hands
    And puts them in her lap *(fold hands in lap).*

Materials: Small objects cut from paper, such as star, ball, and apple (page 29), Masking tape, Tissues

5. Now, we are going to play a game. Try to follow my directions. *Give each child an object cut from paper with a piece of tape on the back.* Listen to my directions. Ready?

    Place the star on your chin.
    Place the apple on your shirt, and then stand up.

    Give each child a paper cut-out plus a tissue. Can you follow my directions? Listen.

    Put the star on the floor and the tissue on your head.
    Continue giving directions that require two actions.

Materials: Variety of classroom objects, such as block, ball, and book

6. *Place objects on table for children to choose from.* We are going to play a game. You must listen carefully and follow my directions. Please choose one thing from the table. *Give each child a direction to follow, such as:*

 ____________________, put your block under your chair.

 ____________________, give your ball to____________________.

 ____________________, put ____________________'s book under the table.

 Each child should have the opportunity to follow directions. Now, listen carefully while I tell you to do two different things.

 Give each child a two-part direction, such as:

 ____________________, give your ball to ____________________, and put____________________ 's doll under the table.

7. We are going to play a guessing game. I am going to give someone a direction to act out. Please guess what that person is doing. *Show children how to play the game by acting out a two-part direction for them to identify.*

 Allow each child to play individually by whispering a command, and then act it out, such as:

 Do a little dance, and then make a funny face.

8. I have a finger play to teach you. It is called "Come, Kitty, Come."

 Come, Kitty; come, Kitty *(motion to come),*
 Here's milk for you *(cups hands for a dish and extend).*
 Kitty came running *(run fingers up arm)*
 And calling, "Meow, meow."

9. *Ask children to pretend to be animals, or assign animals for them to be.*

We are going to play a game. Listen carefully and follow my directions. We are going to be animals.

Give each child a two-part direction based on their animal, such as:

____________________ is a bunny.

____________________, hop like a bunny and eat your carrot.

PROGRESS CHECK

Materials: Common classroom objects

1. *Give one-part directions, using common classroom objects, for each child to follow. Say:*

Listen carefully while I tell you what to do.

Find a book and bring it to me.

2. *Then, give two-part directions for each child to follow.*

Now, walk around your chair, and then walk to the bookshelf.

Scoring:

+	Responds correctly with no prompts
0	Fails to respond correctly with no prompts

Primary: Level B

Activity 1: Body Parts

Objective: To name body parts when given function (all parts)

Materials: Ball
Familiar objects that make sounds (cymbals, bells, other noisemakers)

EYES and EARS

1. We are going to play a game with our bodies.

   These are my eyes. Point to your eyes.
   I see with my eyes. What do you see with?

   After correct response, show children a ball, then take it away.

   What did you see?
   How did you see the ball?

2. These are my ears. Touch your ears. I hear with my ears. What do you hear with? Close your eyes. *Ring a bell, hit a cymbal, or close the door.*

   What did you hear? How did you hear it?

   Now, take turns showing us objects and making sounds for us to guess. *Allow each child to take a turn, then hide objects:*

   What did you see? How did you see it?

   Make sounds. What did you hear? How did you hear it?

   I have a riddle for you. *Teach riddle.*

   A pretty song I want to hear,
   So I must listen with my ____________________.
   I want to see the strawberry pies,
   So I must see them with my ____________________.

NOSE and MOUTH

Materials: Objects to smell, such as orange slice, perfume, flower
(CAUTION: Verify that children have no allergies being doing this activity.)

3. This is my nose. Touch your nose. I smell with my nose. What do you smell with? Smell this. *Give each child an object to smell.* What do you smell? What do you smell with?

   This is my mouth. Touch your mouth. I eat with my mouth and talk with my mouth. What do you eat with? What do you talk with? I have some snacks. What do you want to eat? What do you eat with?

4. Let's review our riddle and add some items. Listen.

   A pretty song I want to hear,
   So I must listen with my ________________.
   I want to see the strawberry pies,
   So I must see them with my ________________.
   I want to smell a pretty rose,
   So I must use my pretty ________________.
   I like oranges from the South,
   And I can eat them with my ________________.

HANDS and FINGERS

5. These are my hands. Show me your hands. I use my hands to clap. How do you clap? Let's try clapping our hands. We can also use our hands to wave. How do you wave? Let's wave with our hands.

6. Let's review our riddle and add some items:

   A pretty song I want to hear,
   So I must listen with my ________________.
   I want to see the strawberry pies,
   So I must see them with my ________________.
   I want to smell a pretty rose,
   So I must use my pretty ________________.
   I like oranges from the South,
   I can eat them with my ________________.
   I can wave, I'm sure I can,
   If I just try to use my ________________.
   If I point to the singer,
   I have to use my pointing ________________.

FEET and LEGS

7. These are my legs. Show me your legs. These are my feet. Show me your feet. I use my legs and feet to run. How do you run? What else can you do with your legs and feet?

8. Let's stand and do some things with out legs and feet. Show me how you can use your legs and feet to *walk* in a circle.

Continue with "run," "jump," "kick a ball," "march," "hop," and "jog."

> Now we'll play a game. You'll each take turns being leader. When you are the leader, you will do something with your legs and feet. We must do whatever the leader does. Be sure to watch the leader carefully.

Let's review the riddles we have been discussing the last few days, and add new parts. Listen, and then let's say the riddles together:

A pretty song I want to hear,
So I must listen with my __________________.
I want to see the strawberry pies,
So I must scc them with my __________________.

I want to smell a pretty rose,
So I must use my pretty __________________.
I like oranges from the South,
And I can eat them with my __________________.

I can wave, I'm sure I can,
If I just try to use my __________________.
If I point to the singer,
I have to use my pointing __________________.

I must walk across the street,
So I will use my little __________________.
I want to run with my friend Peg,
So when I run I will use my __________________.

Body Puzzle

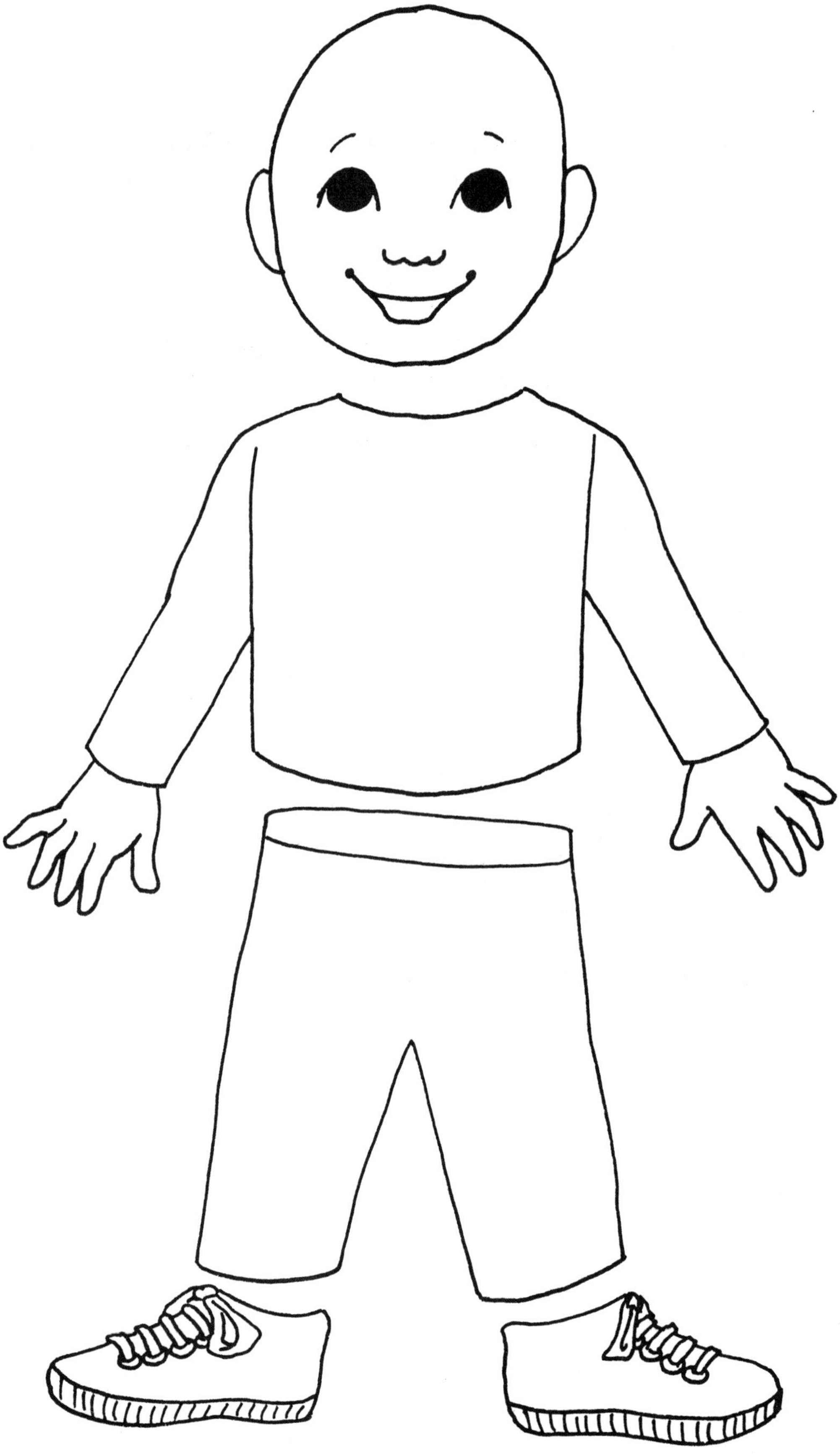

BODY

Materials: Doll or teddy bear
Body puzzle

9. *Review body parts with doll or teddy bear. Introduce body puzzle.* This is a special puzzle of a body. Watch me while I put it together. *Assemble puzzle, naming parts.* Now you try.

Materials: Body puzzle
Flannel board with body puzzle

10. We are going to use the body puzzle. I will give each of you a piece of the puzzle. Help put the puzzle together. First, tell about your puzzle piece, then put it in the puzzle.

    I have a new song. It tells about our body. *Teach song (tune of "Mary Had a Little Lamb").*

    My little feet go
    Run, run, run.
    Run, run, run.
    Run, run, run.
    My little feet go
    Run, run, run.
    They run and
    Run and run.

    Demonstrate actions with the song. Other verses:

    My little ears can hear, hear, hear…
    My little hands can clap, clap, clap…
    My little mouth can chew, chew, chew…
    My little nose can smell, smell, smell…
    My little eyes can see, see, see…
    My little legs can stamp, stamp, stamp…

PROGRESS CHECK

Materials: None

1. What do we see with?
   What do we smell with? Do you talk with your nose or your mouth?
   What do we clap with?
   Tell me what body parts we kick and run with.
   What can we snap?
   What do we hold our pencil with?
   What do we wave with? *Listen.*

2. Place the body part you clap with on the table. What is its name?
   Touch what you smell with. What is it called?
   Tell me what we talk with.
   What do we see with?
   What do we hear with?
   Point to the body parts we run and jump with. What are they called?
   What do we wave with?
   What body part do we see with? *Listen.*

Scoring:

+	Identifies all body parts correctly
0	Fails to identify all body parts correctly

Primary: Level B

Activity 2: Opposites

Objective: To recognize opposites, such as "hot "and "cold," "rough" and "smooth," "hard" and "soft," "wet" and "dry," "sad" and "happy," "fast" and "slow," and "sit" and "stand"

Materials: Objects and pictures to illustrate opposite concepts, such as –

Sand paper and smooth paper
Emery board and tongue depressor
Baseball and sponge ball
Cotton ball and golf ball
Wet washcloth and dry washcloth
Ice cubes and hot soup
Hot water and cold water

HOT and COLD

1. *Put objects on the table that represent the concepts "hot" and "cold."*

   Touch the hot object. This water is hot. Can you find water that is not hot?
   Children locate a cup or glass of cold water. Yes, that water is not hot. The water is cold.
   Call on each child to identify opposites individually.
   Introduce pictures of objects that are hot and cold.
   Have the children select pictures as you say "hot" and "cold."

ROUGH and SMOOTH

2. *Place objects on the table that represent the concepts "rough" and "smooth."*

   Hold up the sandpaper. This paper is rough.
   Can you find the paper that is not rough? *Children locate smooth paper.*
   Yes, that paper is not rough, it is smooth.
   Introduce pictures of objects that are rough and smooth.
   Place pictures or objects used in preceding lessons on the table.

   Let's play the "Opposites" game. Show me the "opposite" of what I pick up. *Pick up an object or a picture.* This paper is smooth. Can you find the paper that is not smooth? Yes, that paper is not smooth, it is rough.

WET and DRY

3. *Put wet and dry washcloths on the table. Touch the wet washcloth.* This washcloth is wet. *Let the children touch the washcloth.* Can you find the washcloth that is not wet?

> *Discuss the opposites "wet" and "dry." Ask the children in turn to locate a wet cloth or a dry cloth. Introduce pictures of "wet" and "dry."* Display one picture from each set of pictures, and put the remaining pictures in a bag. Take a picture from the bag, then see if you can find its *opposite* on the table.

HARD and SOFT

4. *Place hard and soft objects on the table. Hold up the hard ball.* This ball is hard. Can you find the ball that is not hard?

> *Ask the children to locate opposites.* Yes, that ball is not hard; it is soft. *Discuss these concepts. Ask children to find hard and soft objects in turn. Introduce pictures of hard and soft objects. Place all objects or pictures from preceding lessons on table.*

Let's play the "Opposites" game:

> Find the opposite of a hard ball.
> Find the opposite of something hot.
> Touch the opposite of something wet.

HAPPY and SAD

5. *Introduce the opposites "happy" and "sad."*

> I am happy today. Look at my face. *Smile.* How can you tell that I am happy? Yes, I have a smile on my face. Now, I am going to pretend that I just dropped my ice cream cone. I am sad. Look at my face. *Frown.* How can you tell that I am sad? Yes, I am frowning. "Happy" and "sad" are opposites. "Smile" and "frown" are opposites. Now, pretend with me. Show me you are happy. Show me that you are sad.

Introduce pictures depicting "happy" and "sad."

Let's play the "Opposites" game:

> Do the opposite of what I do. Look at me.
> I am sad. Now, show me the opposite.

Opposites

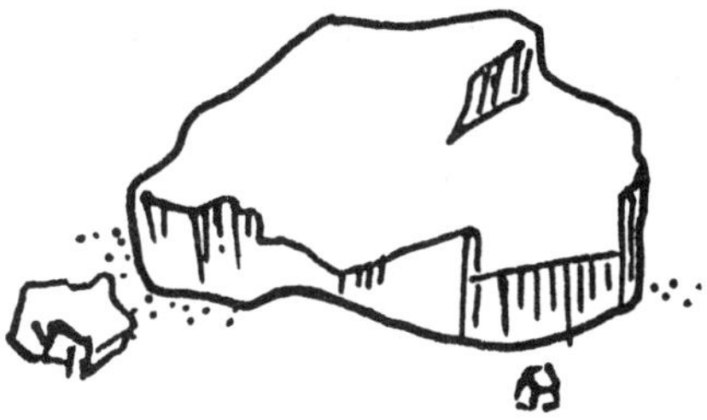

hard

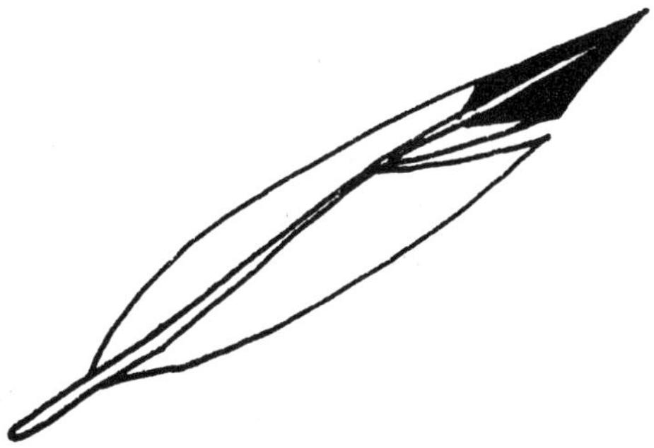

soft

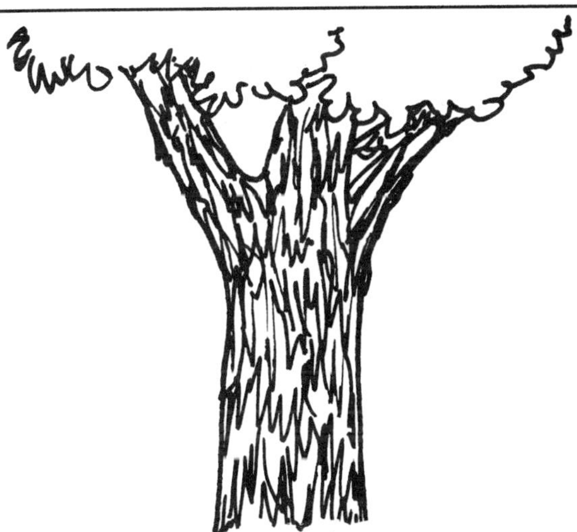

rough

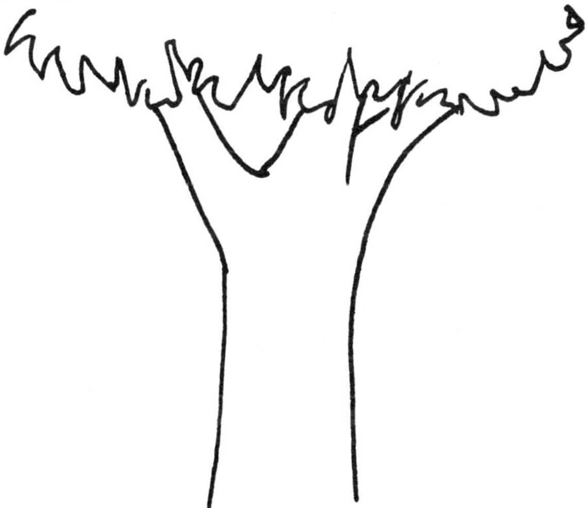

smooth

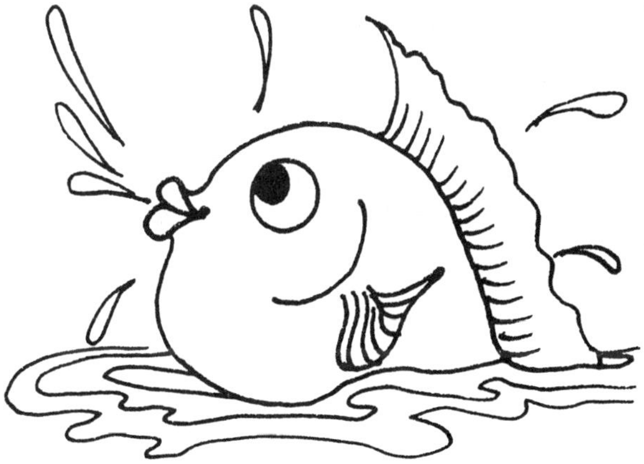

wet

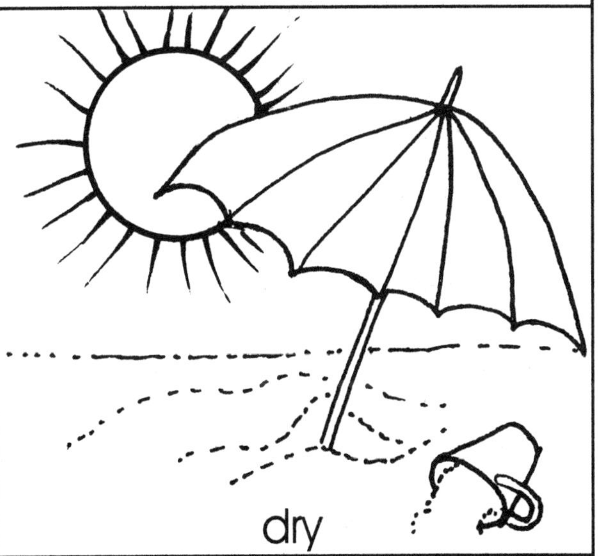

dry

Opposites

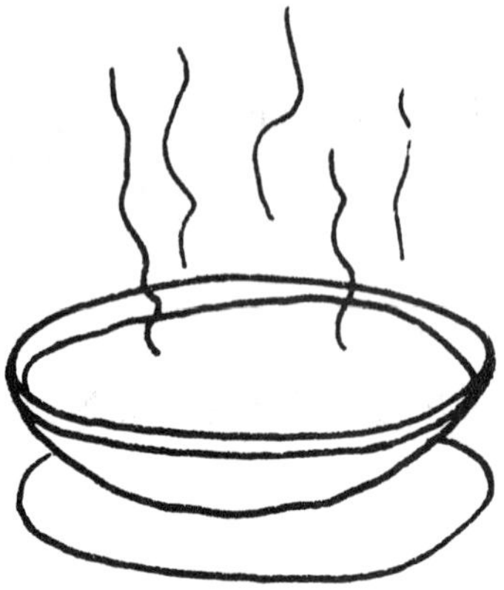

hot

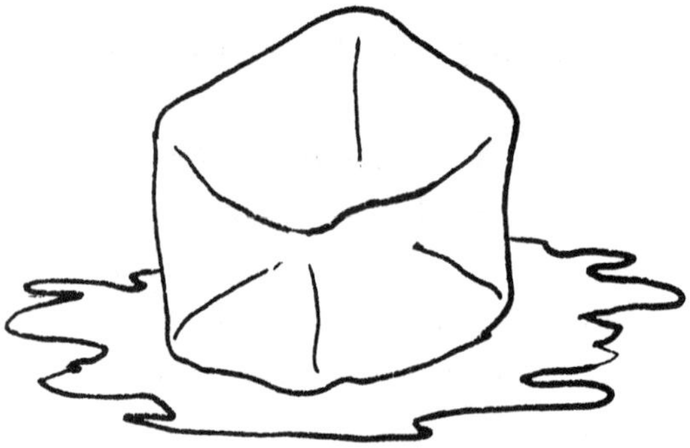

cold

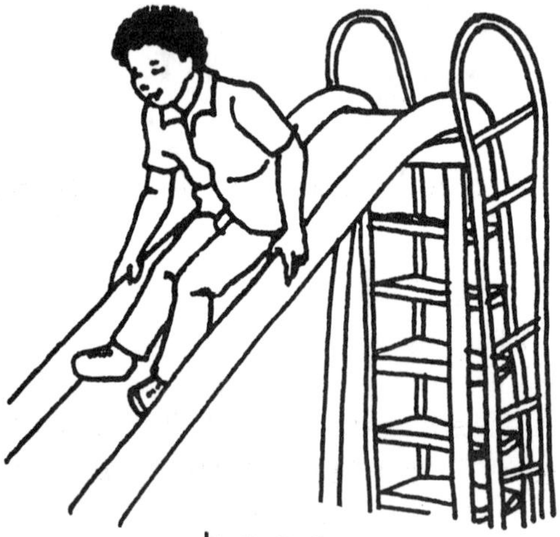

happy

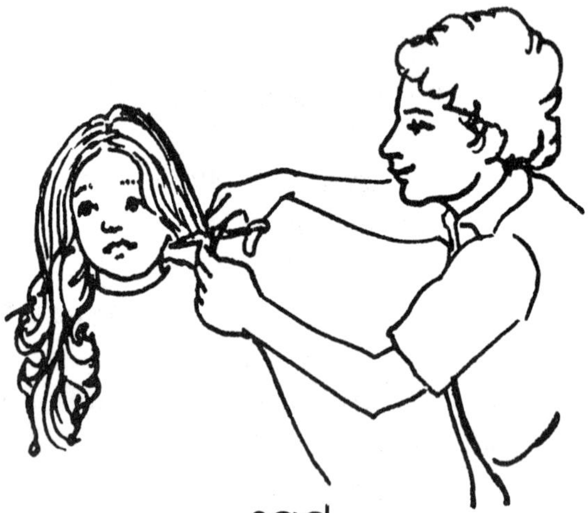

sad

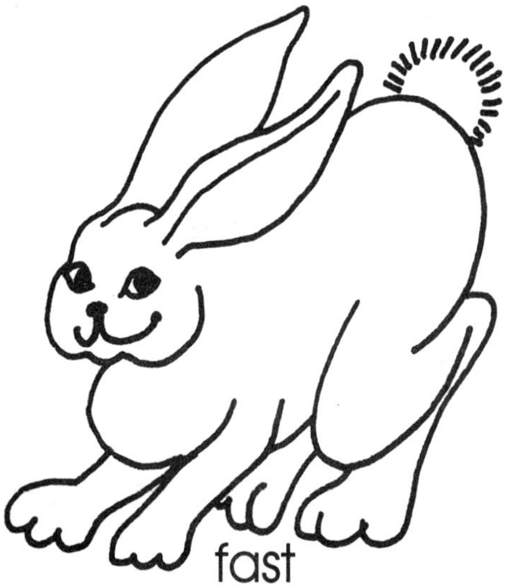

fast

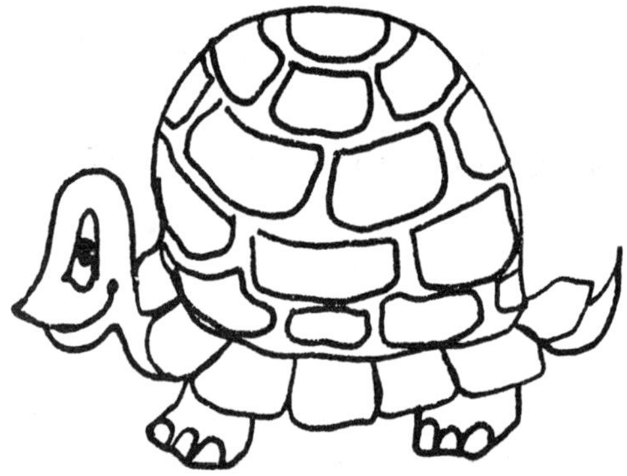

slow

FAST and SLOW

6. Listen carefully. I am going to clap my hands slowly. *Do.* Now, I am going to clap my hands fast.

   "Fast" and "slow" are opposites. Now, listen and do what I say.

      Clap your hands slowly.
      Now, clap your hands fast.

   Let's play the "Opposites" game. I am clapping my hands slowly. *Do.* Now, you do the opposite. Yes, you clap your hands fast.

UP and DOWN

7. Watch me. I am standing up. Now, I am sitting down. Now, you try.

      Stand up.
      Sit down. Good. The opposite of "standing" is "sitting."

   Now, let's try again. When I say your name, you must follow my direction. Ready? *Continue to give directions.*

AWAKE and ASLEEP

Let's pretend. I am going to pretend that I am tired. I am going to sleep. Watch me. Now, I feel rested. I am going to wake up. "Asleep" and "awake" are opposites. Let's pretend we are asleep. Let's wake up and pretend we are awake.

8. We're going to play the "Opposites" game. Whatever I do, you do the opposite. Ready?

      I am sitting down. You must do the opposite.
      That is right, you stand up.

   Now, you be the leader. We will do the opposite of whatever you do.

PROGRESS CHECK

Materials: Objects and pictures to illustrate opposite concepts, such as –

- Sand paper and smooth paper
- Emery board and tongue depressor
- Baseball and sponge ball
- Cotton ball and golf ball
- Wet washcloth and dry washcloth
- Ice cubes and hot soup
- Hot water and cold water

Listen and do what I say:

Put the four sets of objects or pictures on the table. Say: Choose a picture or object. Find its opposite. *Observe.*

Scoring:

+	Chooses all four opposites
0	Fails to choose all four opposites

Primary: Level B

Activity 3: Sentences with Negatives

Objective: To use a sentence pattern with a negative

Using NOT

1. This is not my chin. This is my nose. I am going to point to other places on my body and say part of a sentence. I want you to finish my sentence.

   This is not my foot. This is my ________________.
   This is not my hand. This is my ________________.
   This is not my head. This is my ________________.

   I have a new poem for you. I need your help. When I point to you, I want you to say: "But he wouldn't come out. No, he wouldn't come out." Ready?

   Recite poem to children. Point to children at the refrain for their choral response.

   They Wouldn't Come Out

   I saw a little mouse go into the house.
   I said, "Please, little mouse, come out of that house."

   Refrain:

   But he wouldn't come out.
   No, he wouldn't come out.
   – Beth M. Hui

Materials: Flannel board and felt cut-outs of common objects (page 29)

2. *Place each felt cut-out on flannel board and describe its position using a negative.*

   The star is not at the bottom. It is at the top.
   The apple is not in the corner. It is in the middle.

   Repeat activity. Provide incomplete sentences for the children to finish.

   The circle is not at the bottom. It is at the ________________.

Let's repeat the poem we talked about but add some more to it. Listen.

They Wouldn't Come Out

I saw a little mouse go into the house.
I said, "Please, little mouse, come out of that house."

Refrain:

But he wouldn't come out.
No, he wouldn't come out.

New:

I saw a little hen go into her pen.
I said, "Please, little hen, come out of that pen."

Refrain:

But she wouldn't come out.
No, she wouldn't come out.

New:

I saw a little mole go into his little hole.
I said, "Please, little mole, come out of that hole."

Refrain:

But he wouldn't come out.
No, he wouldn't come out.

New:

So I bought some candy and quick as a dandy,
They all came out; yes, they all came out.
– Beth M. Hui

3. We are going to play a game. It is called "Who Is It?" I will say, "I am thinking of someone who is in this group." Then, I will say, "It is *not* __________________, " and say someone's name. You must say whatever I say. Then, when I say "Who Is It?," tell me who I am thinking of. Ready?

Play game with children by using the pattern sentence:

It is not __________________*(complete the sentence with children's names in turn, omitting the child who is "It"). After each statement, the children repeat,* "It is not __________________."

After all the names but one are called, ask the children: "Who Is It?" *The children respond,* "It is __________________," *naming the person who remains. After a few turns, select a child and say,* Now, you take turns being the leader. You must think of someone, and tell us everyone it is not. Remember, you must say "It is not __________________." Then, call names of those who are not "It." We must say whatever you say. Ready? *Allow each child to lead activity. Praise.*

4. I have a new poem. It is called "What Can It Be?" by Beth M. Hui. *Teach poem.*

There's a strange animal behind that tree,
Oh, what can it be, what can it be?
Is it a bumpy bear?
No, it's not a bumpy bear.
It is a rowdy rat?
No, it's not a rowdy rat.
Is it a lazy ladybug?
No, it's not a lazy ladybug.
Oh, I know!
It's a playful puppy,
And it's mine, all mine.

Materials: If possible, something sweet and something sour for children to taste *(CAUTION: Be sure to check children's allergies before doing activity.)*

5. Let's talk about the things we do and do not like to eat.

First, tell me what you do not like to eat. When I call your name, answer by saying, "I do not like __________________." Then, tell what you do like to eat.

Ask each child to respond.

Materials: Button or other small but *safe* object *(CAUTION: Young children should not be allowed to handle small objects.)*

6. *Put the button in hand and hold hands behind back.*

We are going to play a game called "Which Hand?" I have a button hidden in one of my hands. *Hold hands (closed in fists) in front of you for the children to see.*

I will ask you in turn to guess which hand the button is in.
If you are right, I will say, "Yes, it is in this hand."
If you are wrong, I will say, "No, it is not in this hand."

Ready? *Encourage each child to participate individually.*

Now, you be the leader. I will give you the button to hide. Put it in one hand so we cannot see it. When you are ready, call on different people to guess. Remember, if they are right, you must say, "Yes, it is in this hand." If they are wrong, you must say, "No, it is not in this hand." *Allow each child to lead the game.*

7. *Seat children in a semicircle.* We are going to play a game called, "Listen and Do." I will give you directions. You must follow my directions. Ready? Listen carefully.

Give children actions to perform, such as: Swing your leg.
After a few moments: Do not swing your leg. Wave your arm.
After a few moments: Do not wave your arm.

Continue giving children alternating positive, then negative directions.

Let's play the game again. This time, after I give you a direction, you must say what you are doing. If I tell you to clap your hands, you must clap your hands and say, "I am clapping my hands." If I tell you not to clap your hands, you must not clap your hands and say, "I am not clapping my hands." Ready? Listen carefully.

Continue giving children positive and negative directions. Prompt the children to give complete sentences following the pattern just described.

Materials: Button or other small but *safe* object
Three cups (not transparent)
(CAUTION: Young children should not be allowed to handle small objects.)

8. *Put button under one of three cups.*

We are going to play a game called "Which Cup?" I have a button hidden under one of these cups. I will ask each one of you to guess which cup the button is in. If you are right, I will say, "Yes, it is under this cup." If you are wrong, I will say, "No, it is not in this cup." Ready?

Encourage each child to participate individually.

Now, you be the leader. I will give you the button to hide. Put the button under one cup without our seeing it. When you are ready, call on different people, one at a time, to guess. Remember, if someone is right, you must say, "Yes, it is under this cup." If someone is wrong, you must say, "No, it is not under this cup." *Allow each child to lead game.*

PROGRESS CHECK

Materials: Flannel board and cut-outs
Small but safe objects
Three cups (not transparent)

1. *Place a felt cut-out on the flannel board and describe its position, using a negative sentence. Repeat with three cut-outs. Observe.*

The star is not at the bottom. It is at ________________.

2. I will give you directions to follow. Listen. *Give positive and negative instructions. Observe.*

Clap your hands.	Swing your arm.
Do not swing your arm.	Close your eyes.
Do not close your eyes.	Do not clap your hands.

3. *Introduce buttons and cups. Guess where the button is hidden, then ask the child to respond in a complete sentence. Observe. Continue until the action requires a negative sentence.*

You hide the button under a cup, and I will guess where it is. You tell me if I am right or wrong; remember to use a complete sentence.

Scoring:

+	Uses a complete sentence with a negative
0	Fails to use a complete sentence with a negative

Shapes: Square, Star, and Circle

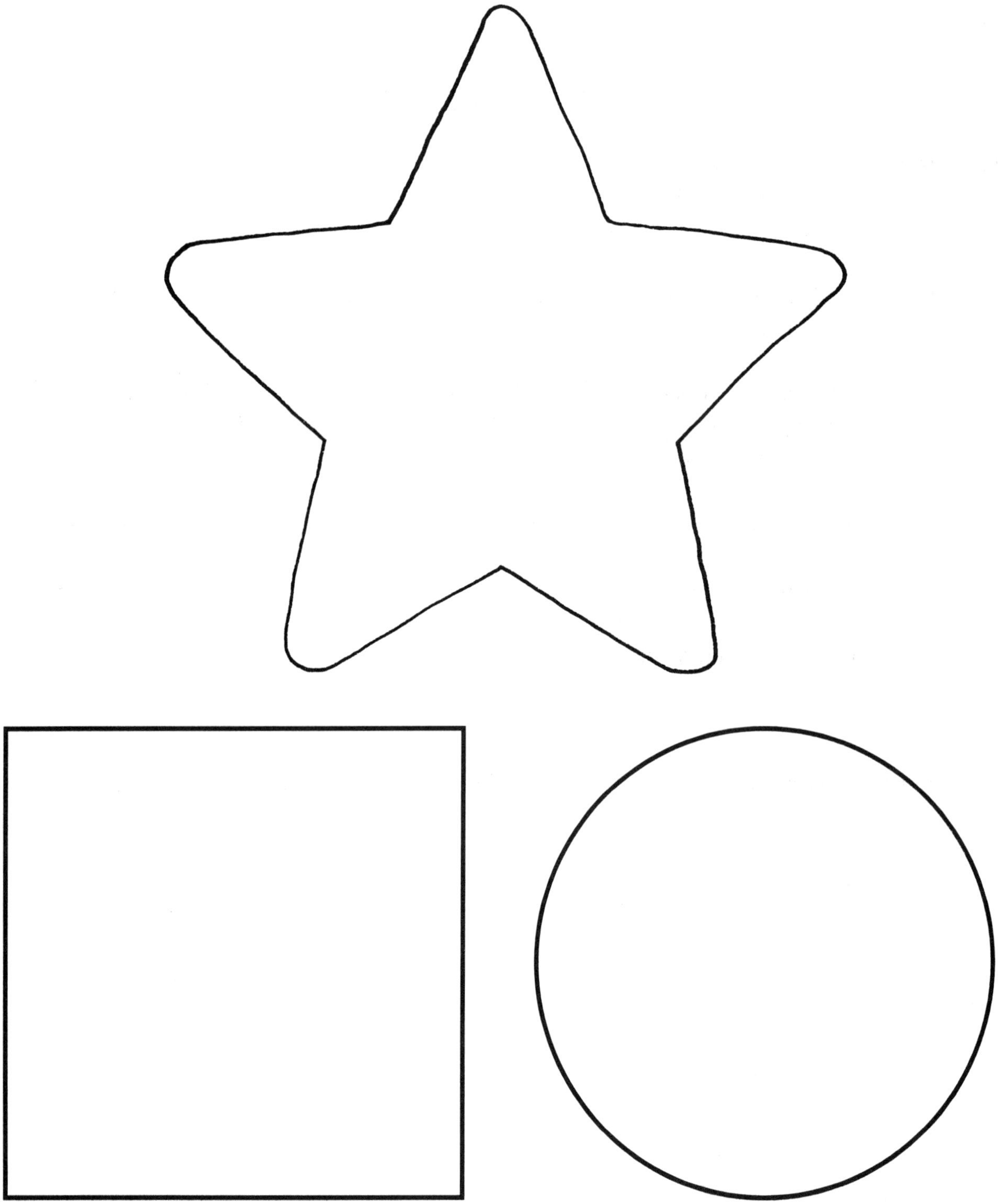

Primary: Level B

Activity 4: Stories

Objective: To tell a story about pictures in sequence

FIRST, NEXT, and LAST

Materials: Wagon or cart
Cereal and bowl
Doll or stuffed animal

1. Watch me. *Put doll or animal in wagon. Pull the wagon. Tip the wagon so the doll falls out. Tell story about action.*

    Look what happened to the doll. I put the doll in the wagon. The doll was riding in the wagon. Suddenly the wagon tipped, and the doll fell out. Watch me again.

    Repeat above action. While the action is occurring, describe what is happening for the children.

    First, I put the doll into the wagon. *Do.*
    Next, the doll went for a ride. *Pull wagon.*
    And last, the wagon tipped over, and the doll fell out. *Do.*

    Allow the children to discuss what happened.

2. *Pour a small amount of cereal into bowl. Sit down and eat it. Tell story describing action.*

    First, I put some cereal into a bowl.
    Next, I ate it.
    And last, the cereal is all gone.
    Now, tell me what I did.

    Demonstrate routine of putting on shoes and socks. Ask one child to take off shoes and socks. __________________ is going to show how to put on shoes and socks. Watch carefully. *Ask the child to demonstrate.* Good.

    Now, tell me what __________________ did first.
    What did __________________ do next?
    What did __________________ do last?

    Direct all questions to all children.

Materials: Small cup
Small blocks
Pictures showing actions

3. Watch me carefully. *Get a cup. Put water in it. Drink the water. Accept and discuss responses.*

   What did I do first?
   What did I do next?
   What did I do last?

   Put small blocks on table. Watch me carefully. *Stack blocks on top of each other until they fall.*

   What did I do first?
   What did I do next?
   What did I do last?

   Show children picture with action.
   Tell what is happening in this picture. *Prompt when necessary.*
   Ask questions to gain more information. Encourage complete sentences. Continue activity with several pictures. Praise responses.

Materials: Box of tissue
Crayons
Paper
Pictures showing action
Flannel board

4. Watch me. *Take a tissue out of the box. Pretend to blow nose. Throw tissue away.*

   What did I do first?
   What did I do next?
   What did I do last?

   Perform another activity: Watch me. *Get crayons and paper. Draw a simple picture; display it on the flannel board.*

   What did I do first?
   What did I do next?
   What did I do last?

   Place action pictures face down on table (enough for each child to have one).
   Choose a picture and tell what is happening in your picture. *Prompt when necessary.*
   Ask questions to gain more information. Encourage complete sentences. Praise responses.

Action Pictures

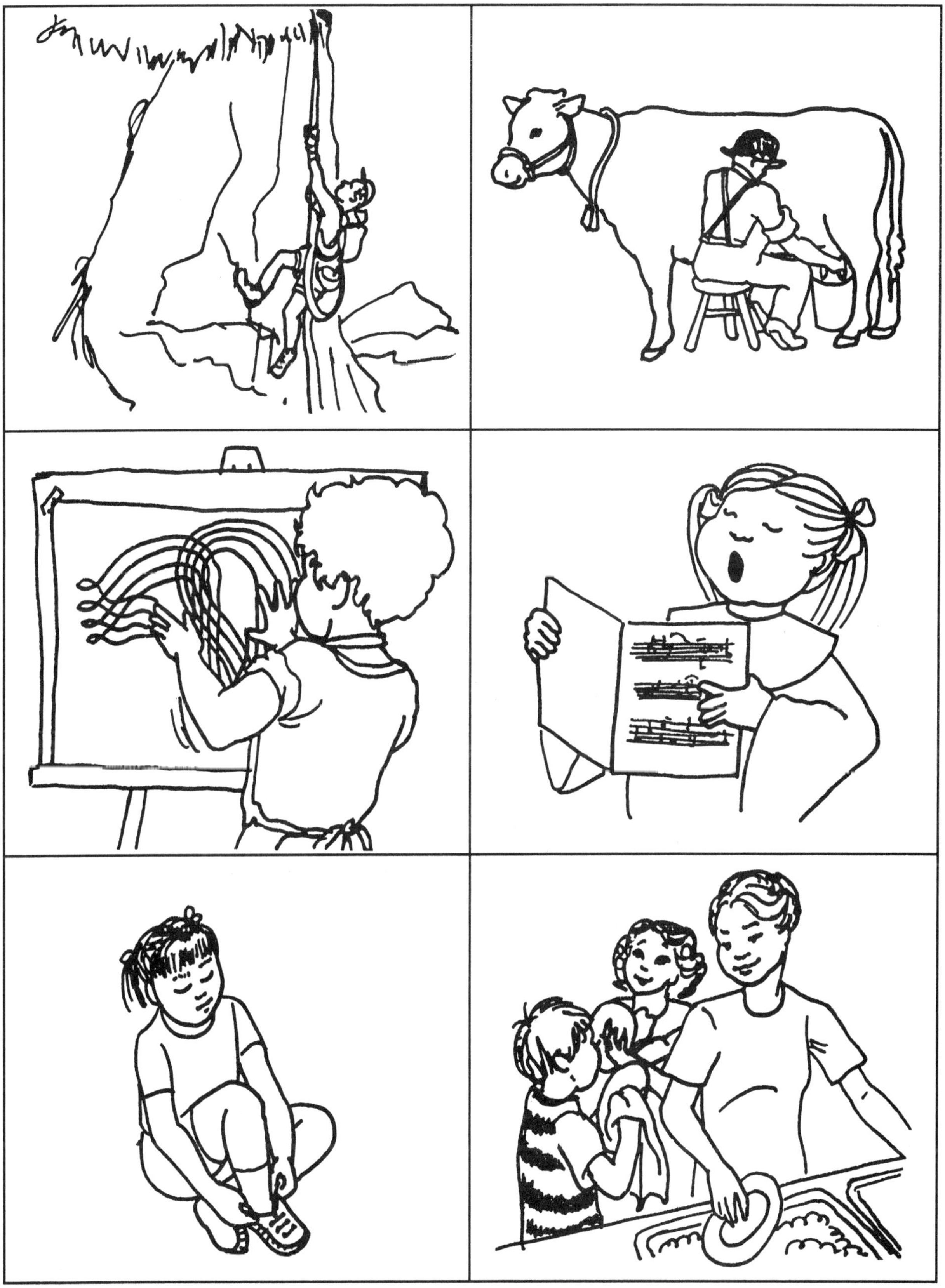

5. *Ask each child to demonstrate familiar routines.* Now, it is your turn to act out something.

   Routines may include:

   Pouring water, then drinking it.
   Blowing nose.
   Building tower of blocks until it falls.
   Drawing a picture for the bulletin board.

   Routines need three distinct actions. Ask:

   What happened first?
   What happened next?
   What happened last?

6. *Put action pictures in bag.* Take a picture from the bag and describe it for us. *Prompt when necessary. Ask questions to gain more information. Encourage complete sentences.*

Materials: At least three sets of three-sequence pictures

7. When I got up this morning, first, I washed my face. Next, I brushed my teeth. Last, I put on my clothes. Tell me what you did first, next, and last this morning. *Prompt when necessary. Ask questions to obtain more information. Encourage use of complete sentences, using "first," "next," and "last."*

8. *Put a set of sequencing pictures on the table. Show children the pictures in sequence. Point to the first picture.* What is happening in this picture?

   Repeat procedure for the remaining two pictures, then give the pictures to the children.

   Who has the picture that comes first? Show us that picture, and tell us about it.
   Who has the picture that comes next? Show us that picture, and tell us about it.
   Who has the picture that comes last? Show us that picture, and tell us about it.

Sequence Pictures: Three Scenes

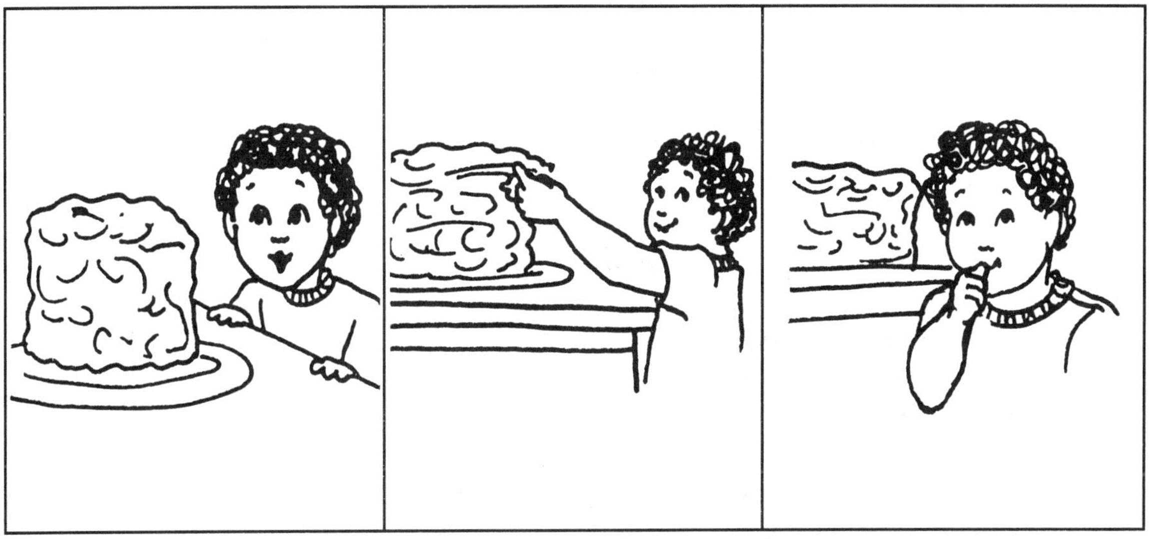

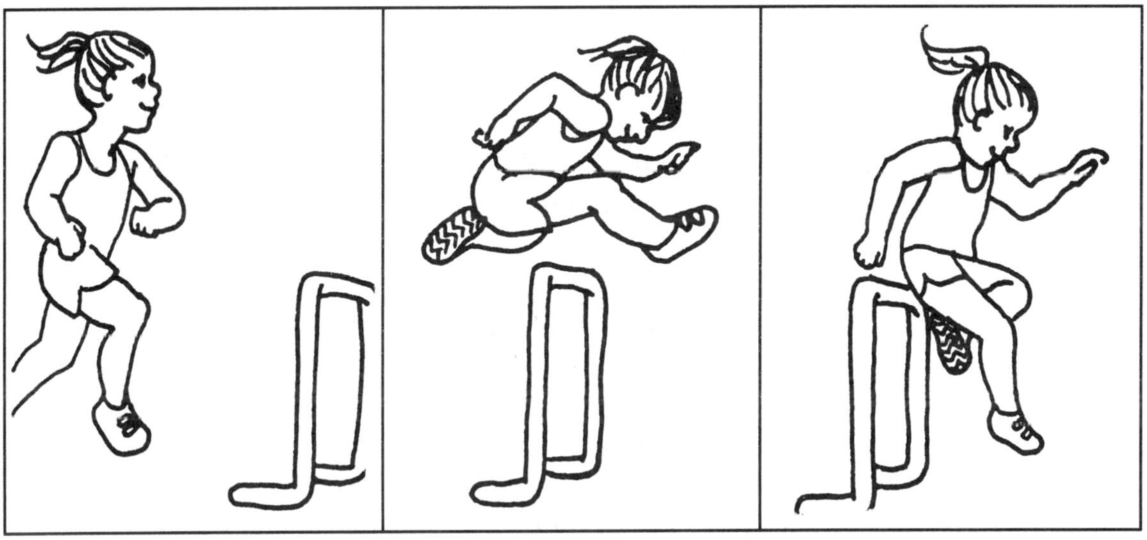

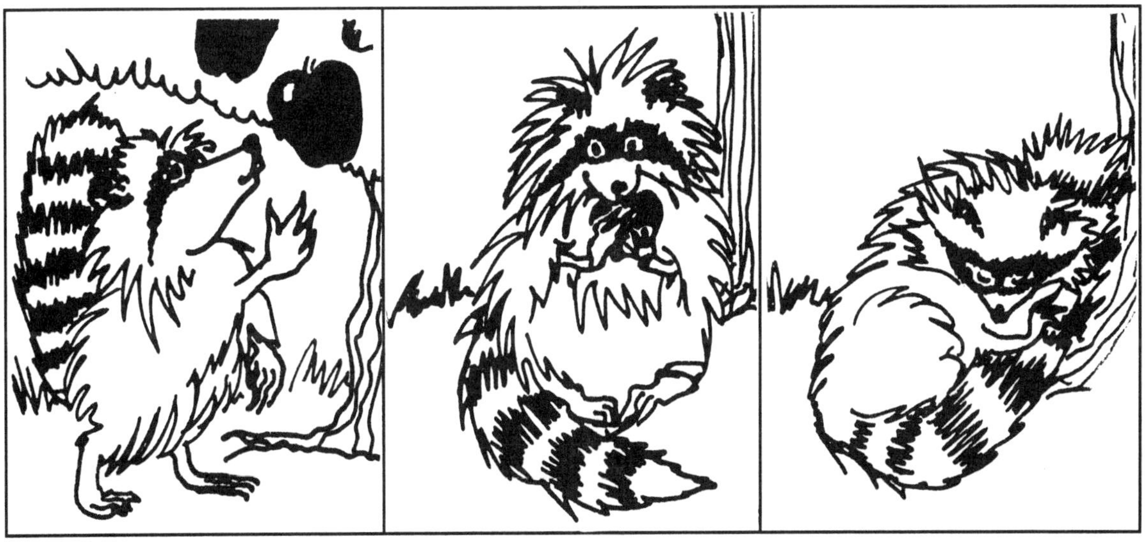

Sequence Pictures: Three Scenes

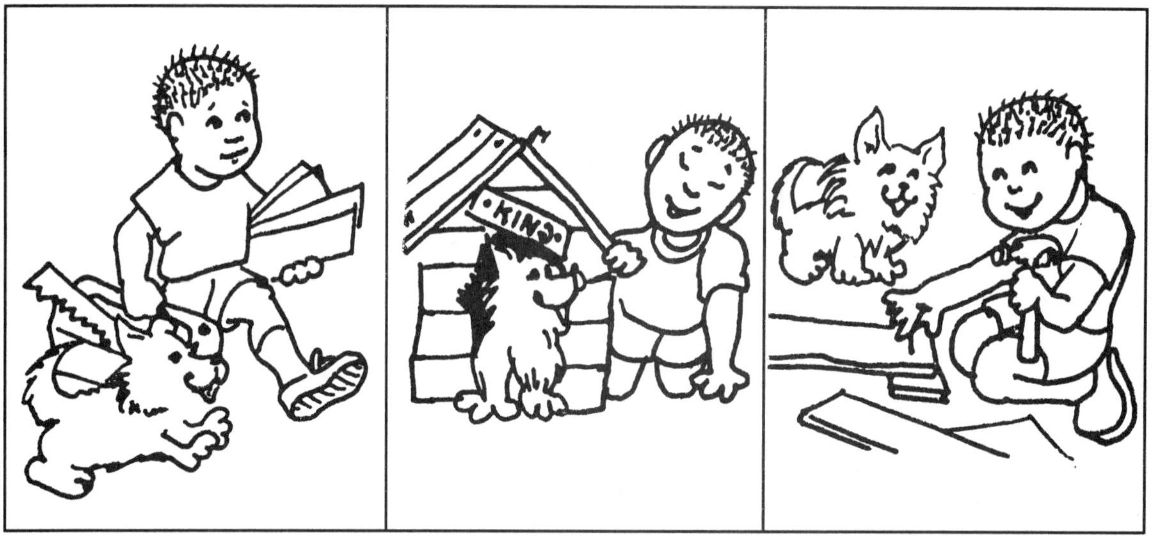

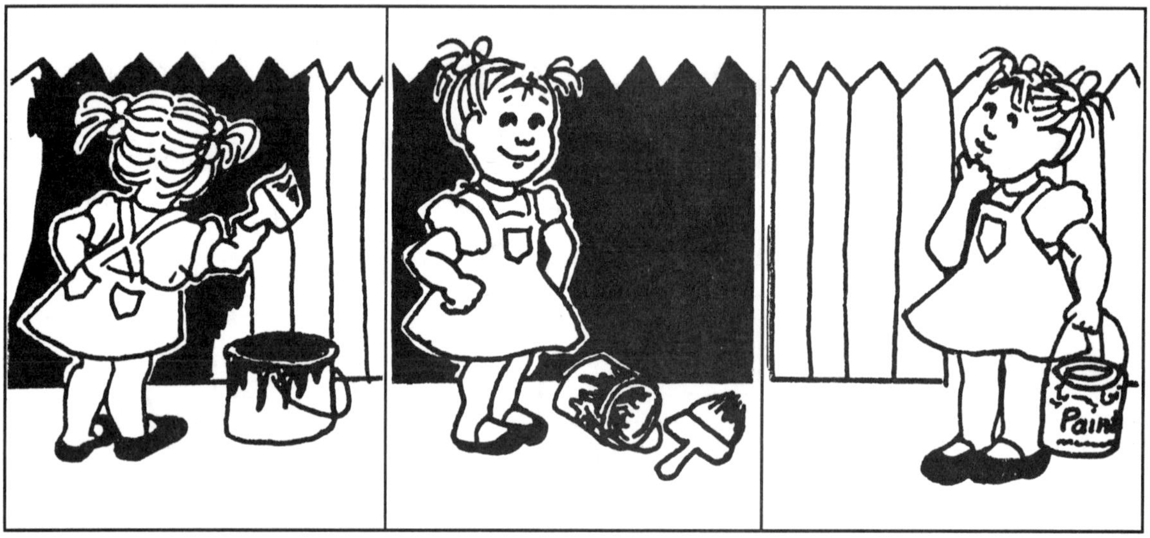

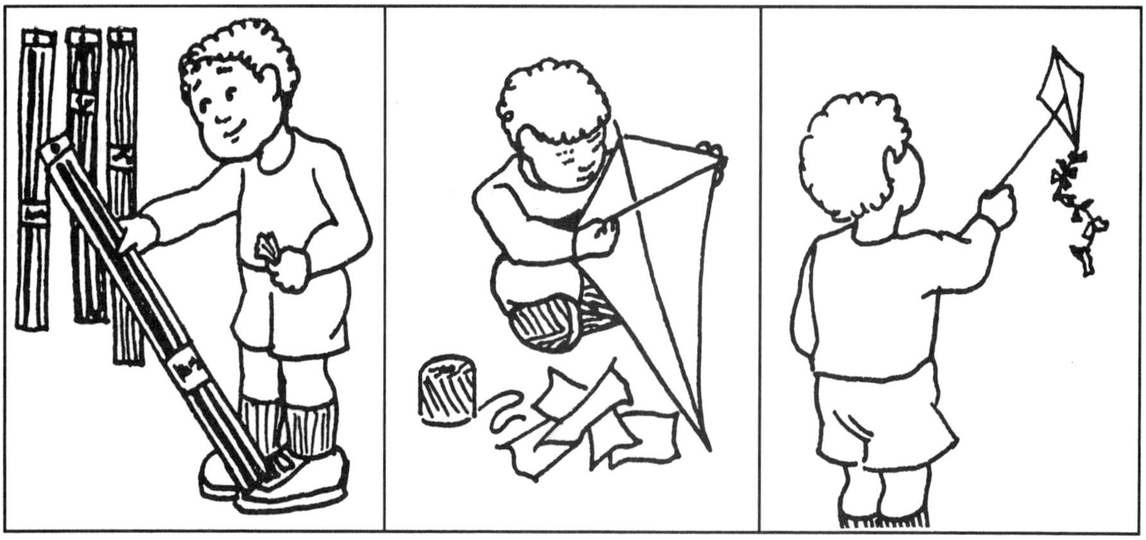

9. *Use one set of pictures. Give a picture to each of three children. Ask children to describe picture (not in order).*

Show us your picture. Tell us what is happening.

When all three have finished:

Which picture comes first? Which comes next? Which comes last?

Ask children to place pictures on the table in correct order. Continue with other sets of pictures. Allow each child an opportunity to participate.

10. I have a finger play to share. *Teach "Jack-in-the-Box."*

This is Jack *(left hand in fist with thumb extended)*
In a box *(put thumb in fist; cover with palm of other hand).*
Open the lid *(lift covering hand);*
Out Jack pops *(pull thumb out of fist with a jerk).*

Discuss finger play. What happened first? What happened next? What happened last?

11. *Give each child a set of pictures to sequence. Say:* Put your pictures in order. *When the child is finished, ask another child to describe the pictures, using words "first," "next," and "last."*

_________________, tell us about _________________'s pictures.

PROGRESS CHECK

Materials: At least three sets of three pictures each that can be sequenced ()

Give child a set of pictures to sequence. Put your pictures in order; tell me about them, using the words "first," "next," and "last." *Observe.*

Scoring:

+	Sequences and describes pictures, using "first," "next," and "last"
0	Fails to sequence and describe pictures correctly

Primary: Level B

Activity 5: Main Idea

Objective: To recall the main idea of a simple story

Materials: Two or three large pictures depicting actions

1. *Show children a picture. Tell them a simple story about it.*

    This is a picture of a girl. She was running. She fell down and hurt her knee. Her mother put a bandage on it for her.

    What is this story about?
    What happened to the girl?

    Encourage the use of complete sentences. Continue activity with other pictures.

Materials: Illustrated nursery rhyme book

2. Let me read a rhyme to you. *Choose an action rhyme to read, while showing picture.*

    What is this rhyme about?
    What happened?

    Continue with several rhymes, allowing each child the opportunity to participate. Now, when I read the rhyme, you act it out. *Select children to demonstrate the actions in the rhyme.*

3. I have a poem to share. Listen carefully. *Recite "My Little Kitten."*

    My little kitten ran up a tree,
    And sat on a limb to look at me.
    I said, "Come, Kitty," and down he ran,
    And drank all the milk I poured in the pan.
    – Beth M. Hui

    What happened in this story?
    What did the little kitty do?

    Encourage the children to respond in complete sentences. Teach the poem to the children. Allow them to act it out.

4. *Show children action pictures. Tell a simple story. For example, show a picture of a woman driving (page 75) and tell this story.*

> This woman is going to the store. She is going to buy food for her family. She is going home now.

What is the story about? What happened to the woman? *Encourage children to use complete sentences and give a simple summary.*

5. I have a poem to share. *Read:*

> The eency, weency spider went up the water spout.
> Down came the rain and washed the spider out,
> Out came the sun and dried up all the rain.
> The eency, weency spider went up the spout again.

Other suitable poems include "'Way Down South" by Withers and "There Was a Little Turtle Who Lived in a Box" by Vachel Lindsay. *After each poem, ask:* What is this about? *Praise actions and responses.*

Story Picture

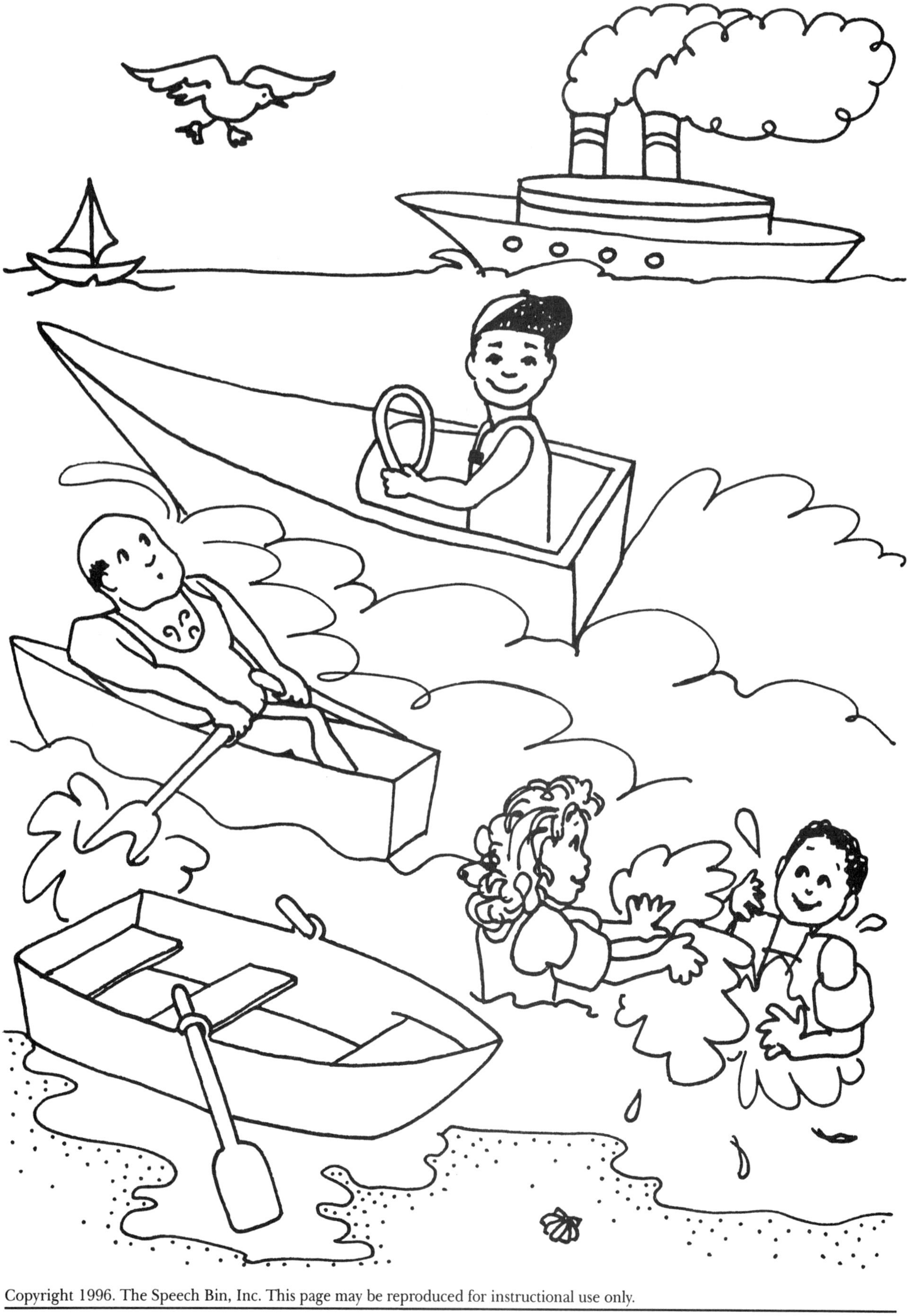

Story Picture

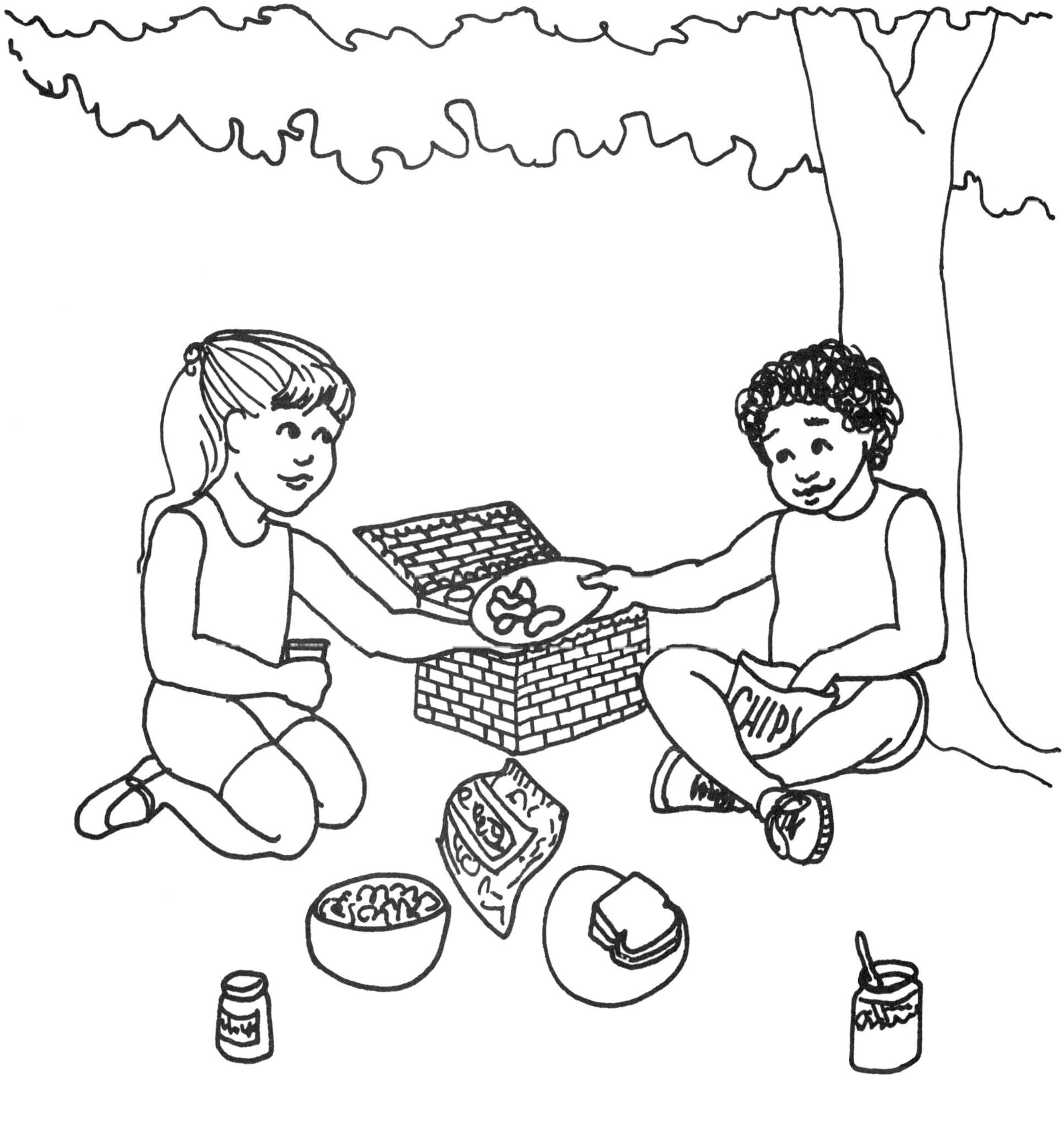

PROGRESS CHECK

Materials: Action pictures

1. *Put action picture on table. Tell the child short (four or five sentence) story about the picture:*

   Listen carefully while I tell you a story about this picture.

   Now, you tell me what my story was about. *Prompt child once if necessary.* What happened in the story? *Observe.*

2. Listen carefully while I tell you a story. *Tell child short (four or five sentence) story.*

   The little boy wanted to go outside and play. He went to the closet, got his sweater, and put it on. Then, he told his mother we was going outside to play. When he opened the door to go outside, he saw it was raining.

   Now, tell me what my story was about.

Scoring:

+	Summarizes story without any prompts
0	Fails to summarize story without any prompts

Action Pictures

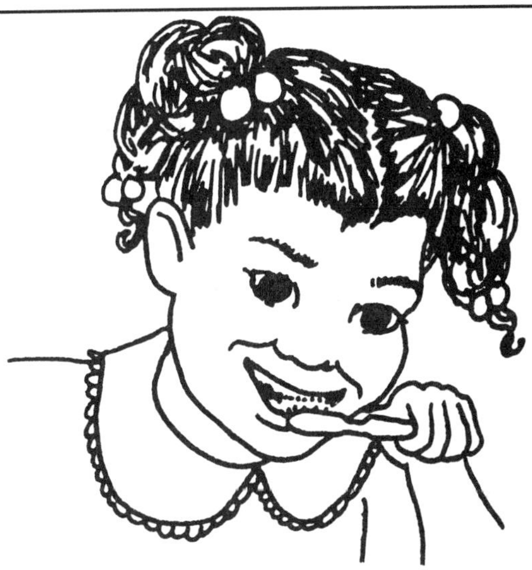

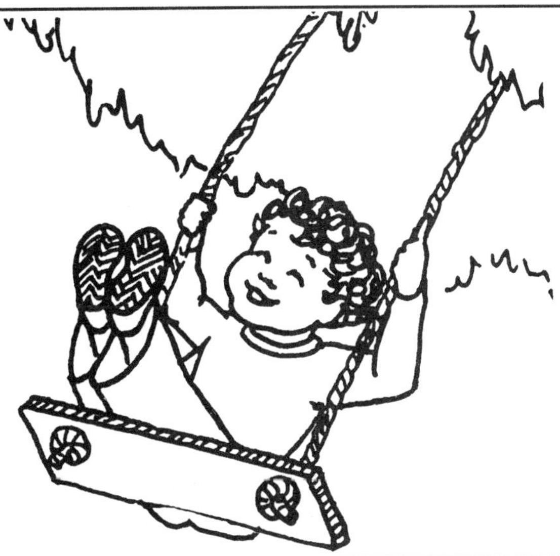

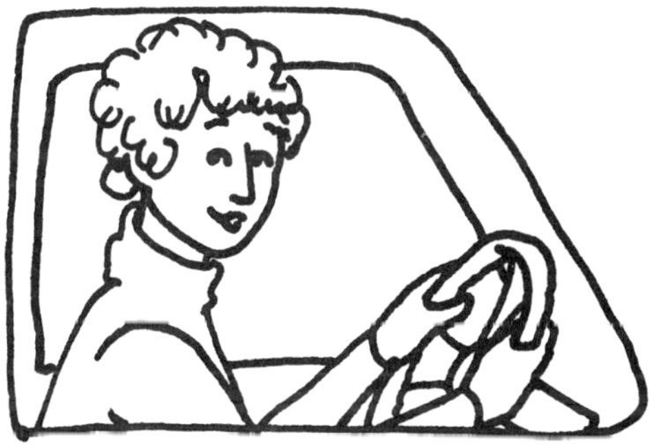

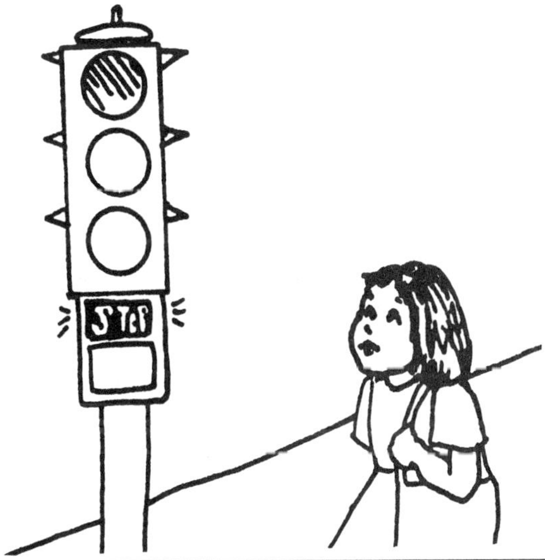

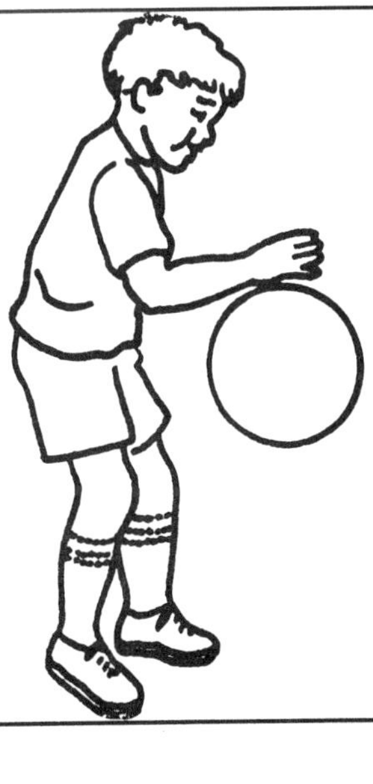

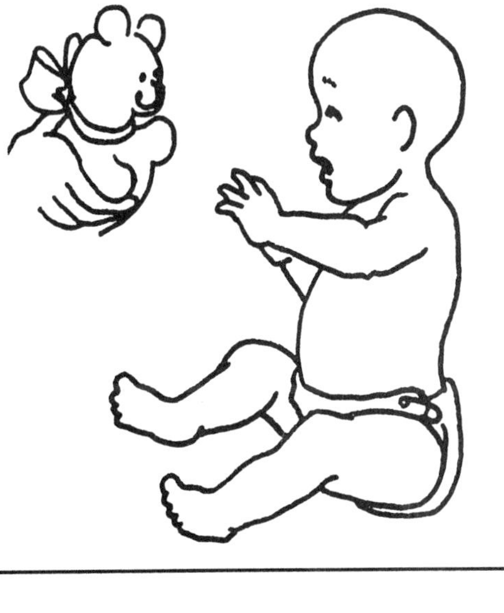

Intermediate: Level C

Activity 1: Functions of Objects

Objective: To express function of familiar objects

Materials:
Ball
Cup
Shoe

1. *Display materials. Hold up the cup.*

   What is this? Yes, it's a cup.
   What do we do with a cup? Yes, we drink with it.
   What are other things we can use to drink with?

   Encourage discussion of objects used for drinking. Continue activity for ball and shoe. Discuss uses of ball, such as throwing, kicking, and bouncing. Discuss why shoes are worn.

   I have some riddles to share. Try to guess these riddles. *Recite riddles.*

   You pour milk in me to fill me up,
   You use me to drink from. I'm a ________________.

   I'm always round; sometimes big, sometimes small.
   You can bounce me and throw me. I'm a ________________.

   I come in different colors; sometimes old, sometimes new.
   Just put me on your foot and wear me. I'm a ________________.

Materials:

Cup	Fork
Spoon	Scissors
Shirt	Sock
Shoe	Coins
Pen and pencil	Bag

2. *Place objects in bag. Select one object from the bag. Ask children in turn to select object.*

   What is it?
   What is it for?
   What else can we do with it?

3. I have some riddles to share. Try to guess my riddles. *Recite riddles:*

Fry some bacon if you can.
Use me to cook with, I'm a ________________.

Let's take a trip near or far.
You can ride in me, I'm a ________________.

"Go to sleep," your mother said.
Lie down on me, I'm a ________________.

I have words and pictures; just take a look.
Your teacher can read me, I'm a ________________.

Materials:

Cup	Fork
Spoon	Scissors
Shirt	Sock
Shoe	Coins
Pen	Pencil

Action pictures, such as –
eating, counting money, cutting

4. Let's play a game called "Match Me." I will give each of you an object. Then, I will hold up a picture. If the picture goes with your object, say, "Match Me." Ready?

Give each child an object, then hold up action pictures. Prompt when necessary, so each child will be successful.

5. Let's go for a walk. Follow me. *Lead children on walk around the room. Point to familiar objects and ask their functions. Point to a chair.* What is this? Yes, it is a chair. What is it for? What other things do we sit on? *Continue with other objects using same procedure.*

Materials:

Cup	Fork
Spoon	Scissors
Shirt	Sock
Shoe	Coins
Pen and pencil	Bag

6. *Display materials. Review the name and function of each object with children.*

Let's play a game called "What Is It?" I am going to describe an object. You must tell me what it is. Ready? *Ask all children to respond.*

I'm thinking of something you eat with. What is it?

Action Pictures

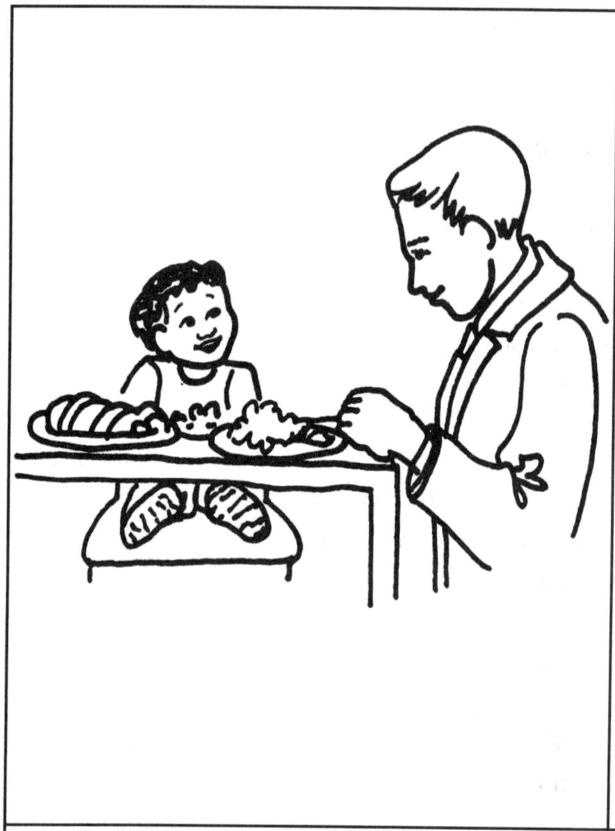

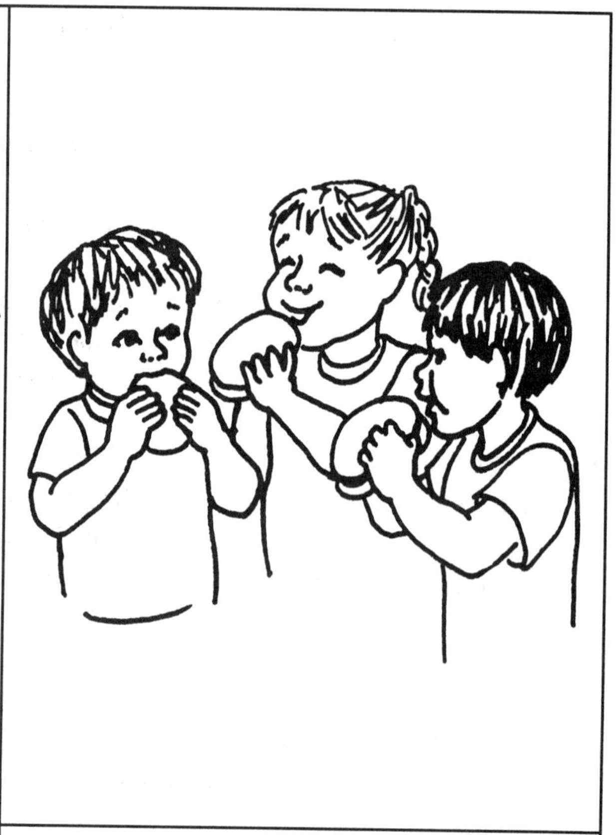

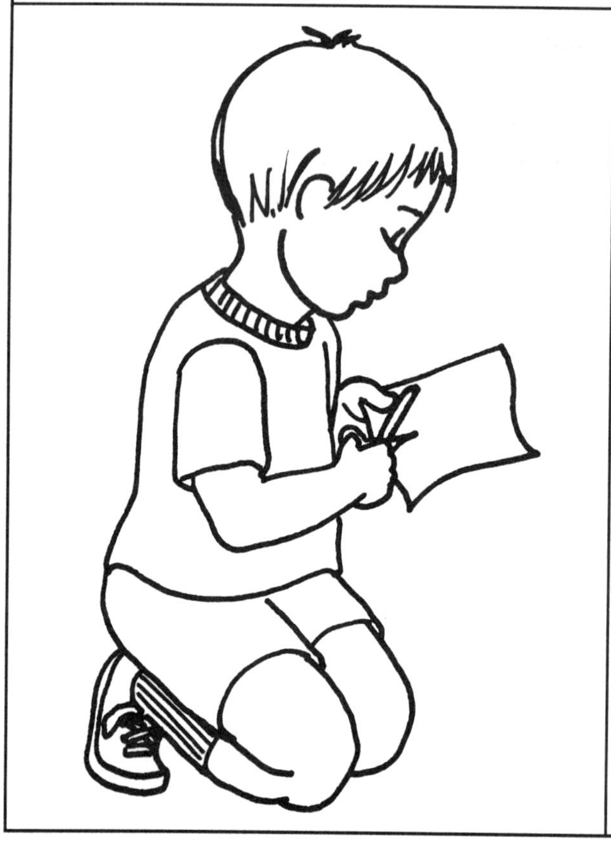

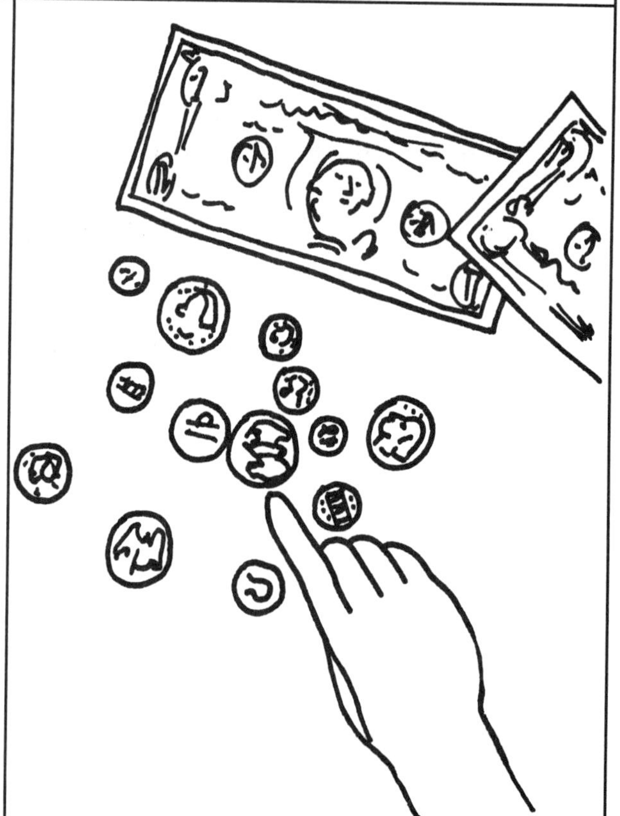

Materials: Pictures of familiar objects (such as bed, cup, ball)

7. *Place pictures face down on table.* Let's play a game. When I call your name, pick one picture. Show us your picture. Tell us what it is and what it is used for. Ready? *Ask each child to answer questions.*

 ____________________, choose a card. Show us your card. What is it?

 Yes, it is a bicycle. What is it used for?

 Yes, a bicycle is to ride. What else can we ride? *Continue activity, giving each child opportunity to participate. Prompt when necessary. Praise responses. Repeat activity with different sets of pictures.*

8. Let's play a new game called "Name It." Try to name as many objects as you can that are used for the same thing. Ready? Name things that you wear. *Hold up fingers as children name items that can be worn. When finished, say:* You named things we can wear. *Continue activity with other categories, such as things to play with or things to write with.*

9. *Place pictures in bag. Take one picture from the bag. Tell what it is and what it is for. Let each child participate. Prompt with questions when necessary. Place same pictures on table, face up.* Look at the pictures. I'm thinking of something to sleep on. What is it? *After correct response, remove pictures. Continue activity until all pictures have been used.*

10. *Review pictures by discussing their names and uses. Then, place pictures face down on table.*

 Please choose a picture. Don't show it to anyone, and don't tell what it is. Instead, tell what you do with it. Watch me and listen.

 Select a picture. This is something that ____________________ *(tell its use).*

 Ask: What is it? *Provide more clues if necessary. Give each child an opportunity to participate in turn. Prompt when necessary. Repeat activity, using different sets of pictures.*

Objects: Ball, Bicycle, Broom, Glass, Bed, Comb

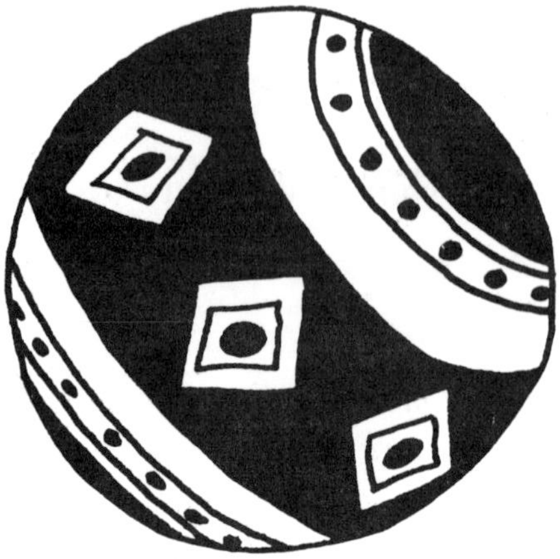

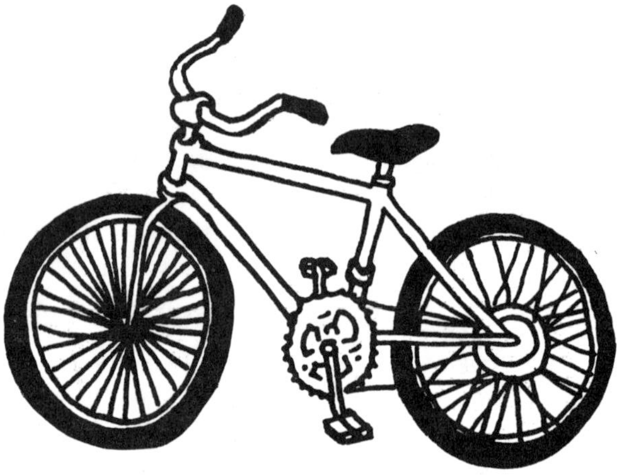

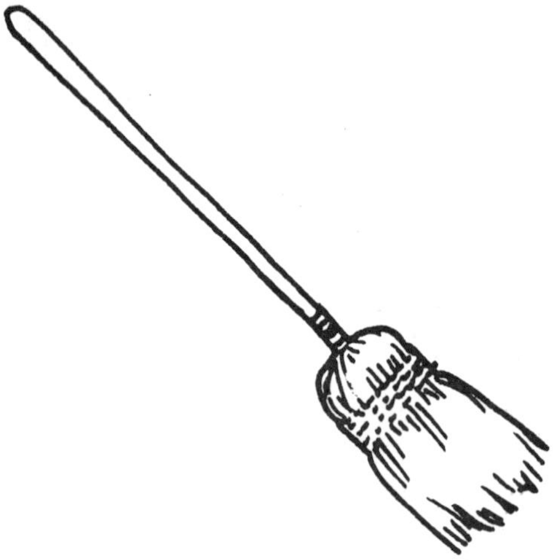

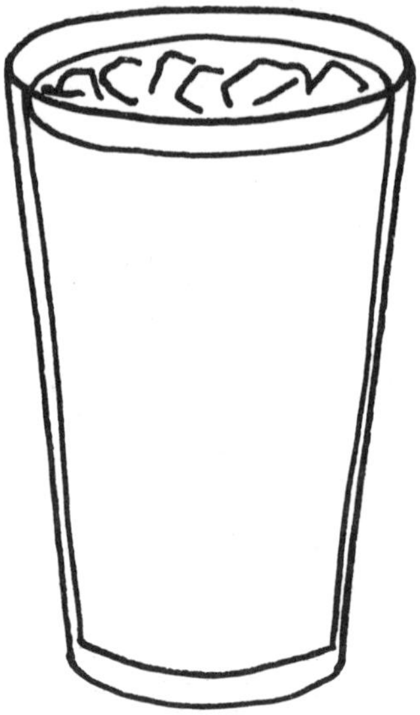

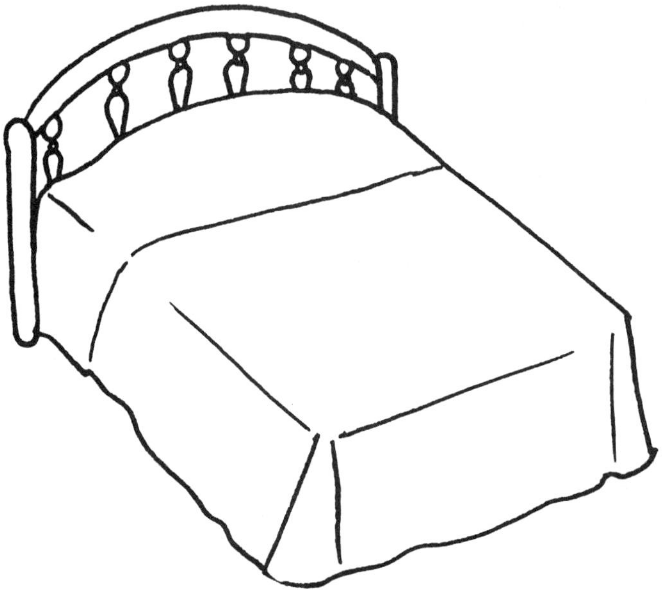

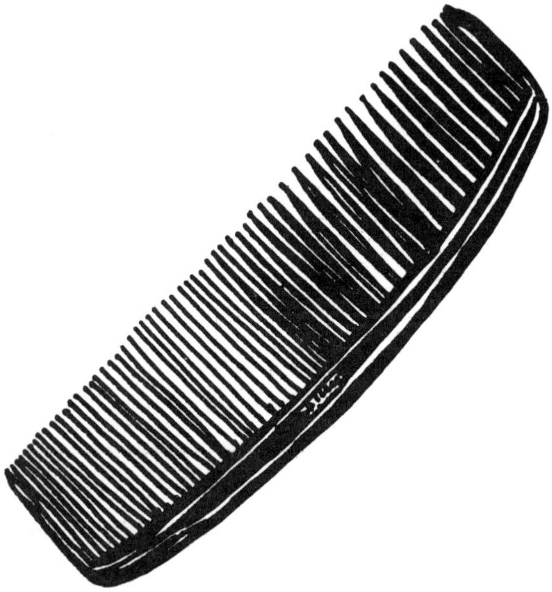

Objects: Baseball, Cup, Shoe, Fork, Spoon, Scissors

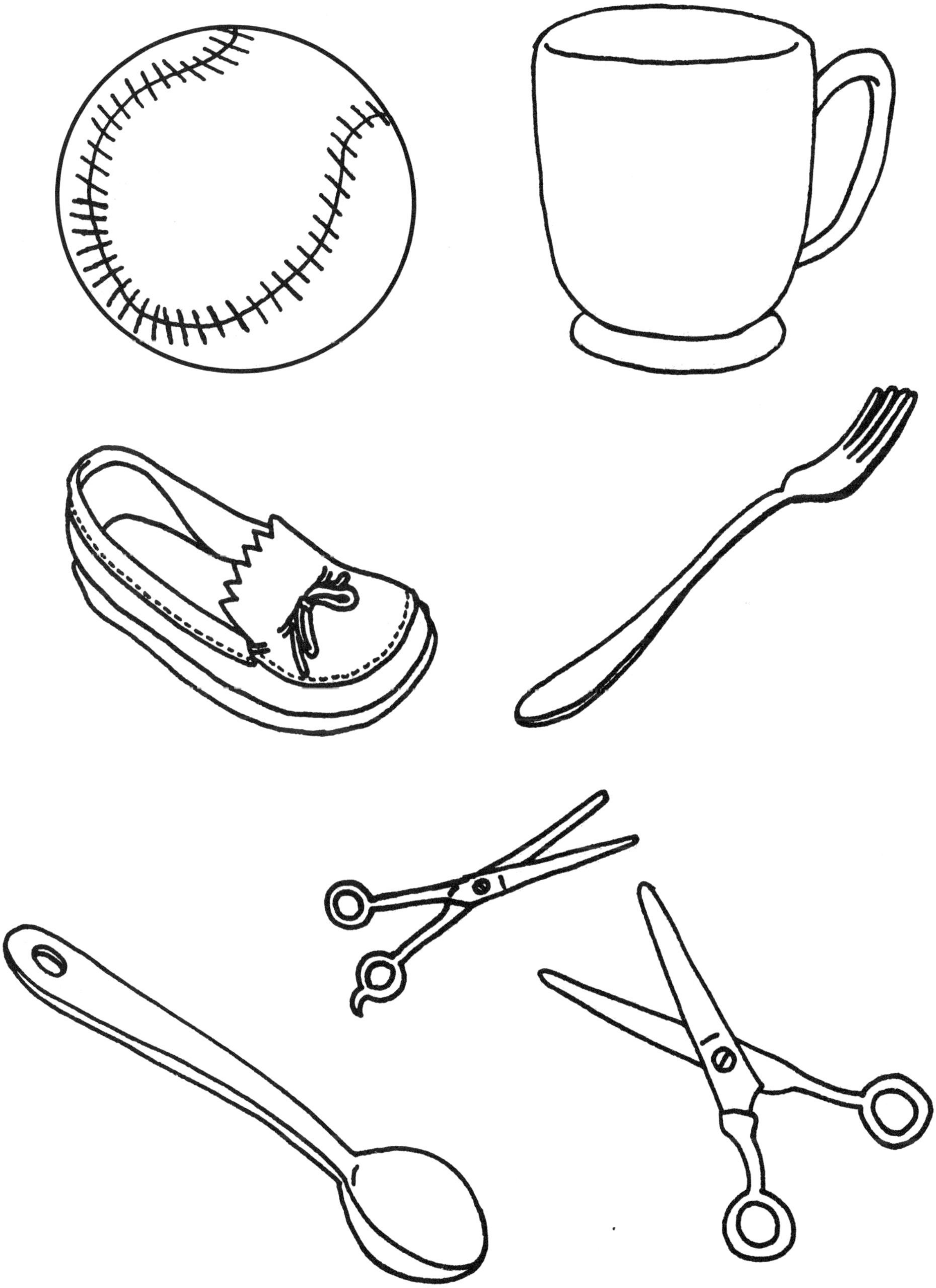

PROGRESS CHECK

Materials: Pictures of familiar objects or the objects themselves (used previously) –

Cup	Fork
Spoon	Scissors
Shirt	Sock
Shoe	Coins
Bag	Pen and pencil

1. *Take an item from the bag and say:* "What is this? What can we do with it?" *Continue until all items have been used. Observe.*

2. *Show children objects or pictures of objects. Ask them to name and give the functions of five objects or pictures.*

Scoring:

+	Names and expresses function of five objects or pictures
0	Fails to name and express function of each object or picture

Intermediate: Level C

Activity 2: Naming Colors

Objective: To name colors (red, yellow, blue, orange, green)

Materials: Colored blocks or beads (five of each: red, yellow, blue, orange, and green)

1. *Display red and blue blocks. Say:*

   These blocks are alike except for color. Some blocks are red, and some blocks are blue.

   Display a blue sheet of paper. Hold up a blue block.

   Find a block exactly like this one, then put it on this sheet of paper.

   Ask children in turn to select one blue block and put it on the blue sheet of paper. Put red and blue blocks together. Put red sheet of paper in place of blue sheet. Repeat above activity, asking children in turn to select block exactly like your block (red), and place it on the sheet of red paper. Display all blocks.

   I've added another group of blocks. They are alike except for color. Some blocks are red, some blocks are blue, and some blocks are yellow.

   Display a yellow sheet of paper. Hold up yellow block.

   Choose a block that looks just like this and put it on this sheet of paper.

   Continue until all blocks have been placed.

Materials:

Five red blocks	Five blocks of other colors
Five red objects	Five objects of other colors
Red badges (red paper circles with tape on the back)	

2. *Display all blocks; review colors.* What makes these different? Yes, their color. *Hold up a red block.* This is a red block. Find another red block. *Let children answer individually. Display all objects (not blocks). Hold up red object.* What color is this?

   Yes, it is red. It is a red ________________ *(name object).* Find something else that is red. Tell what it is.

   Hold up a red badge. This is a red badge. *Put a red badge on each child.* Please find one object that is red like your badge, then bring it to us. *When children return, review objects.* This is a red ________________ *(name object).*

Materials: Five blue blocks | Five blocks of other colors
Five blue objects | Five objects of other colors
Blue badges (blue paper circles with tape on the back)

3. *Display all blocks.* What makes the blocks different? Yes, their colors make them different.

Hold up a blue block. This is a blue block. Find another blue block. *Allow each child to select a blue block. Display all objects (not blocks). Hold up blue object.*

What color is this? Yes, it is a blue ________________ *(name object).*
Find something else that is blue. Tell us what it is.

Hold up blue badge. This is a blue badge. *Put a blue badge on each child.* Please find one object that is blue like your badge, then bring it to us.

After children finish, review objects. It is a blue ________________ *(name object).*

Materials: Five blue objects | Five red objects
Bag | Red and blue sheets of paper

4. *Display all objects. Hold up a red object.*

This is a red ________________ *(name object).* Can you find a red object? *Allow each child to select a red object. Regroup objects. Repeat above procedure for blue objects. Put all objects in bag. Display red and blue sheets of paper.*

Let's play a game. Pick one object from the bag. Tell if it is red or blue, then put it on the red or blue piece of paper. Watch me.

Select an object from the bag. Identify its color and place it on the appropriate sheet of paper. Display all objects, mixed for color.

Let's play a game called "I Spy." I will choose one object and describe it to you. Try to guess what it is. Ready?

I spy with my little eye something blue. What is it?

Give all children the opportunity to guess. Further clues may be given for specific objects. When object is identified, remove it and continue.

Materials: Five yellow blocks — Five blocks of other colors
Five yellow objects — Five objects of other colors
Yellow badges (yellow paper circles with tape on the back)

5. *Display all blocks; review colors with children.*

What makes the blocks different? Yes, it is their color.

Hold up a yellow block. This is a yellow block. Find another yellow block.

Display all objects (not blocks). Hold up yellow object. What color is this?

Yes, it is yellow. It is a yellow ____________________ *(name object).* Find something else that is yellow. Tell us what it is.

Hold up yellow badge. This is a yellow badge. *Put a yellow badge on each child.*

Please find one object that is yellow like your badge, then bring it to us.

When children return, review objects. This is a yellow ____________________ *(name object).*

Materials: Five orange blocks — Five blocks of other colors
Five orange objects — Five objects of other colors
Orange badges (orange paper circles with tape on the back)

6. *Display all blocks; review colors with children.*

What makes the blocks different? Yes, it is their color.

Hold up an orange block. This is an orange block. Find another orange block.

Display all objects (not blocks). Hold up orange object. What color is this?

Yes, it is orange. It is an orange ____________________ *(name object).* Find something else that is orange. Tell us what it is.

Hold up an orange badge. Say: This is an orange badge. *Put an orange badge on each child.*

I want you to walk around the room and find one object that is orange like your badge, then bring it to us.

When children return, review objects. This is an orange ____________________ *(name object).*

Materials: Five green blocks
Five blocks of other colors
Five green objects
Five objects of other colors
Green badges (green paper circles with tape on the back)

7. *Display all blocks; review colors with children.* What makes the blocks different? Yes, it is their color.

   Hold up a green block. This is a green block. Find another green block.

   Display all objects (not blocks). Hold up green object. What color is this? Yes, it is green. It is a green __________________ *(name object).* Find something else that is green. Tell us what it is.

   Hold up green badge. This is a green badge. *Put a green badge on each child.*

   Please find one object that is green like your badge, then bring it to us.

   When children return, review objects. This is a green __________________ *(name object).*

Materials: Large color cards of red, orange, yellow, blue, green*
Pictures of objects, such as food, clothing, toys
Pictures of objects to color
Red, yellow, orange, blue, and green crayons

* *To make color cards, glue colored construction paper to index cards or laminate construction paper.*

8. *Hold up a red color card.* This color is red. If you are wearing red, stand up.

   After response: Look around the room. What do you see that is red?
   After response: Can you think of something outdoors that is red?

   Use the same procedure with yellow, orange, green, and blue color cards. Then, show children the pictures of objects; describe these objects and their colors.

   This is a red apple.

   After pictures are discussed, lay them face down. Say: Choose a picture, and tell about it.

   Allow each child to select a picture and describe it. Praise. Give children crayons (one of each color) and pictures to color. Hold up a red crayon.

   What color is this?
   What things on your paper could be red?
   Yes, the apple is red. Color your apple red.

   Continue with the other colors.

Objects: Red, Orange, Yellow, Blue, Green

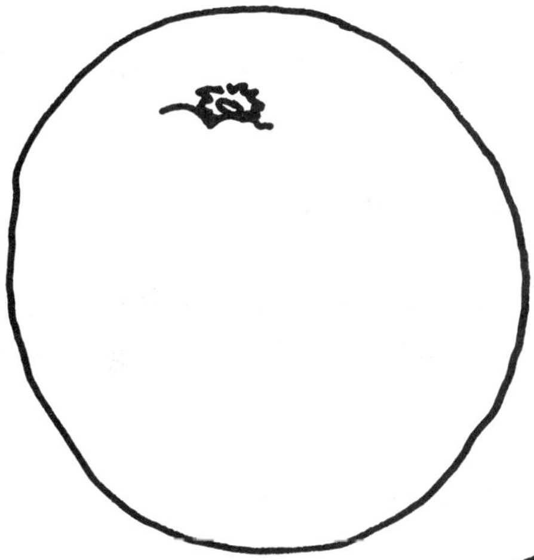

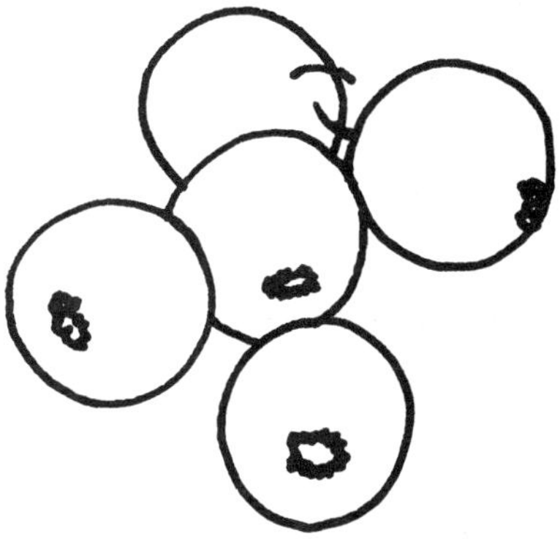

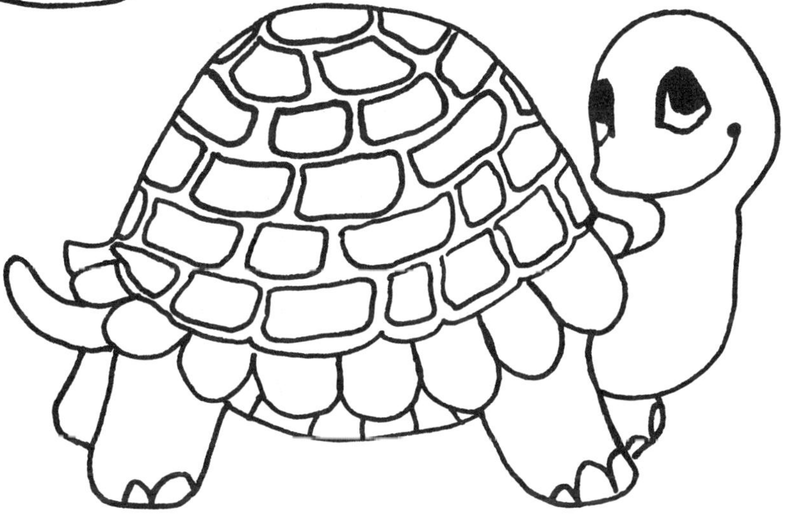

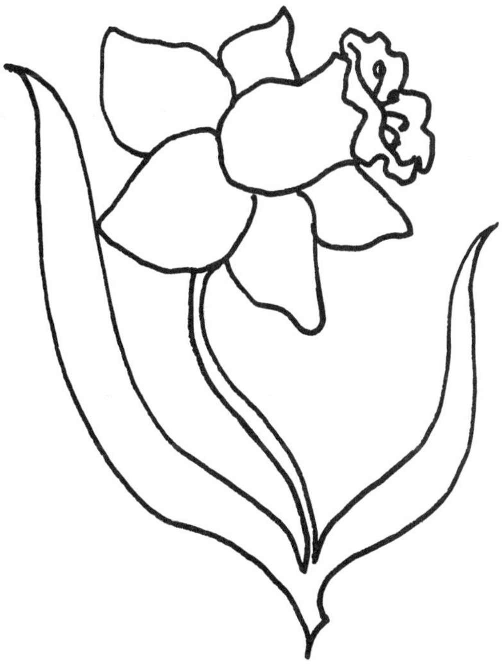

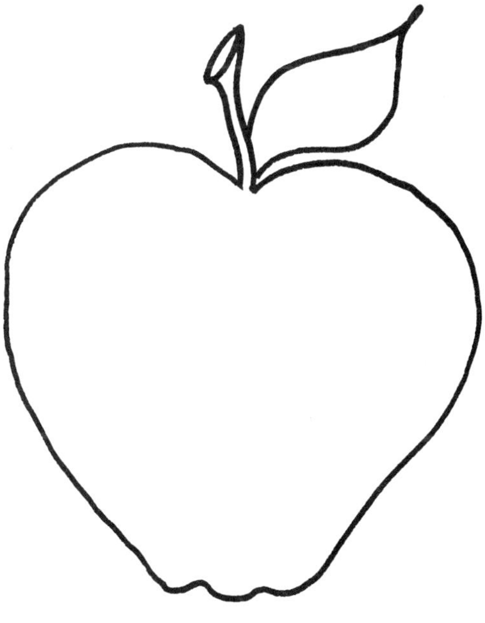

PROGRESS CHECK

Materials: Colored blocks (five of each color: red, yellow, blue, orange, and green)

Display blocks, objects, and crayons on the table, making sure two or three of each color (red, yellow, green, blue, and orange) are shown.

Ask each child to select all objects that are the same color as the piece of paper displayed, and then name the color.

Repeat this procedure until all have been selected and their colors named. Observe.

Scoring:

+	Selects objects and names that color for all five
0	Fails to select objects of same color and name all five colors

Instructional: Level C

Activity 3: Sentences

Objective: To use a sentence pattern with past tense and/or a function word

1. *Introduce self to children.* My name is Ms./Mr. ________________. Please say your name, using a complete sentence. Say, "My name is ________________," then say your name.

   Ask all children to tell their names, using complete sentences.

   Now, let's tell how we came to school this morning. I'll go first. I came to school in a car. ________________, how did you come to school?

   Encourage use of complete sentences. If a child answers with one word ("car," for example), say: You rode in a car. Good. Now say, "I rode in a car."

   I have a rhyme to share. *Recite:*

   Jack and Jill went up the hill
   To fetch a pail of water.
   Jack fell down and broke his crown,
   And Jill came tumbling after.

   Ask questions:

   Where did Jack and Jill go?
   What happened to Jack?

Materials: Large bag
Empty boxes and cans of food (or pictures of foods, found on page 33)

2. Let's take a shopping trip. *Display bag filled with empty boxes and cans (or pictures) of foods.*

   Let's pretend we've been to the grocery store. Pick an object from the bag, and tell what you bought at the store. I'll go first.

   Choose an item from bag; show it to the children. Say: I bought some cereal. Now, you try.

   Allow each child to select and describe an item, using the pattern, I bought ________________. *Encourage use of complete sentences.*

   If a child answers with one word (for example, "orange"), *say:* Yes, you bought an orange. Now you say, "I bought an orange."

3. I have a rhyme to share. *Teach.*

    Hickory, dickory, dock.
    The mouse ran up the clock.
    The clock struck one,
    The mouse ran down,
    Hickory, dickory, dock.

    Ask: Where did the mouse go? What struck one? Then, what did the mouse do? *Encourage use of complete sentences.*

4. *Give each child a simple action to perform.*

    ____________________, open the door. What did you do?

    Child responds: I opened the door.

    Continue activity, giving each child several opportunities to participate. If a child answers with a word or phrase, encourage use of complete sentences. Prompt if necessary.

5. I have a rhyme to share. *Teach.*

    Humpty Dumpty sat on a wall.
    Humpty Dumpty had a great fall.
    All the king's horses and all the king's men
    Couldn't put Humpty Dumpty together again.

    Ask: Where did Humpty Dumpty sit? What happened to him? Who tried to help Humpty Dumpty? Did they help him?

Materials: Toys, such as ball, wagon, doll, blocks

6. *Give children in turn simple actions to perform with toys.*

    ____________________, please stack these blocks.

    When completed, ask: What did you do?

    Continue the activity, encouraging children to answer in complete sentences, using past tense (for example, "I stacked the blocks.") Then continue, adding directional prepositions (such as "under," "between," "beside"). Praise responses.

    ____________________, roll the ball under the table.

    When completed, ask: What did you do?

Encourage children to answer in complete sentences, using past tense and preposition. For example, "I rolled the ball under the table."

Continue the activity, asking other children to describe actions:

__________________, kick the ball into the corner.

__________________, what did __________________ do?

Children respond by naming child and action, using past tense and preposition:

__________________ kicked the ball into the corner.

Materials: Familiar objects, such as book, eraser, doll
Box

7. *Gather items from the room and place them in box.*

I need your help to put all these objects in the box in their correct places.

Give each child directions in turn:

__________________, please take the book to the bookcase.

When the task is completed, ask group: What did __________________ do? *Encourage children to complete sentences with past tense.*

__________________took the book to the bookcase. *Respond:* Yes, she took the book to the bookcase.

Continue until each child has had an opportunity to participate.

8. I have a rhyme to share. *Teach.*

Little Miss Muffet sat on her tuffet
Eating her curds and whey.
Along came a spider and sat down beside her
And frightened Miss Muffet away.

Ask: Where did Miss Muffet sit? What was she doing? Who sat down beside her? What did she do then? *Encourage children to use complete sentences with past tense.*

Stars

Materials: Paper stars Masking tape

9. *Place tape on backs of paper stars so they will stick to objects. Show children the stars. Say:*

Please put the star somewhere on your body.
Then, I will ask someone else to tell me where your star is. Watch me.

Put star on arm. Ask each child: ___________________, where did I put my star?

Encourage children to answer in complete sentences with past tense. Say:
You put the star on your arm.

If a child responds with one word, assist in forming complete sentences. Respond:
Yes, I put the star on my arm.

Give each child opportunity to participate.

Materials: Flannel board
Felt cut-outs of shapes (such as apple, banana, star)
Yarn

10. *Form circle on flannel board with yarn. Place the star in the circle.*

I am putting the star in the circle. ___________________, where did I put the star?

Encourage use of complete sentences. You put the star in the circle.

Respond to child's statement. Yes, I put the star in the circle.

Now, I am going to put the apple on top of the board. *Place apple.*
Where did I put the apple?

Encourage use of complete sentences. You put the apple at the top of the board.
Respond to the child's statement. Yes, I put the apple at the top of the board.

Continue procedure using other cut-outs, giving each child opportunity to participate. Praise.

Now, you try.

Allow children to place a cut-out on flannel board. Ask:
Where did ___________________ put the banana?

Encourage use of complete sentences as outlined above.

PROGRESS CHECK

Materials: Toys, such as ball, wagon, doll, blocks

Using objects, perform simple action, such as putting a ball on the table. What did I do?

Perform three actions. Observe.

Scoring:

+	Performs and responds
0	Fails to perform and respond correctly to all actions

Materials: Flannel board
Cut-outs
Yarn

Use yarn to make a circle on the board. Display cut-outs.

Put a cut-out on the flannel board, then tell me where you put it.

Ask each child to place three cut-outs on the flannel board, then tell where they were placed, using past tense. Observe and listen.

Now, you tell me what I have done.

Scoring:

+	Responds in complete sentences, using past tense
0	Fails to respond in complete sentences, using past tense

Intermediate: Level C

Activity 4: "Wh-" Questions

Objective: To respond to "wh-" questions

Materials: Paper and pencil Illustrated book of nursery rhymes

1. *Give each child simple tasks to do.*

 ____________________, please bring me a pencil. I want to write something on this paper.

 After task is completed, ask the group questions about what happened:

 Who helped me? **What** did they get me? **Where** did they get it? **Why** did I need a pencil?

 Encourage use of complete sentences.

Materials: Illustrated books of nursery rhymes

2. *Use a well-illustrated book of nursery rhymes. Read a rhyme, such as "Humpty Dumpty." Ask children questions about rhyme, such as:*

 Who is this rhyme about? **Where** was Humpty Dumpty sitting? **What** happened to Humpty Dumpty? **Who** tried to help Humpty Dumpty? **Why**?

 Encourage children to answer in complete sentences.

Materials: Toys Illustrated book of nursery rhymes

3. *Put children in pairs and give them simple tasks.*

 Please take these blocks and build a tower. Take turns putting one block on top of another until the tower falls. See how high it can go.

 After task is completed, ask questions about what happened:

 Who built a tower? **What** happened to the tower? **Where** did the blocks fall? **Why** did the blocks fall?

 Give each pair of children an opportunity to participate.

Materials: Items for playing "store" (toys or empty food boxes and cans)
Wagon
Table
Illustrated story "The Three Bears"

4. *Set up items for store.*

Let's go shopping. Let's pretend we're going to the toy (or grocery) store.

Show the children the wagon. We will go to the store in our wagon.

__________________ and __________________, please go to the store first.

__________________, you can take __________________ to the store in the wagon.

When the children take the wagon to the table, ask:

Who is in the wagon? **Who** pulled the wagon?

Ask the children to get a few items, then return them in the wagon.

Ask: **Where** did they go? **Why** did they go? *Encourage use of complete sentences.*

Continue activity, giving children an opportunity to participate in pairs.

After a few times, change items in store (change to toys or food) and vehicle (such as a tricycle).

5. I have a story to share. Please act out the story while I tell it. *Assign parts; set up props. Read "The Three Bears," showing the pictures.*

Who was the little girl? **Where** did she go? **What** did the little girl see in the woods? **Who** lived in the little house? **Why** did the bears go for a walk? **When** Goldilocks got in the house, **what** did she see? **What** did she do? **Why** did the baby bear's chair break? **When** did the three bears come home?

Praise responses. After children discuss the story and its characters, guide them to role play the story, encouraging them to be as creative as they can.

Action Pictures

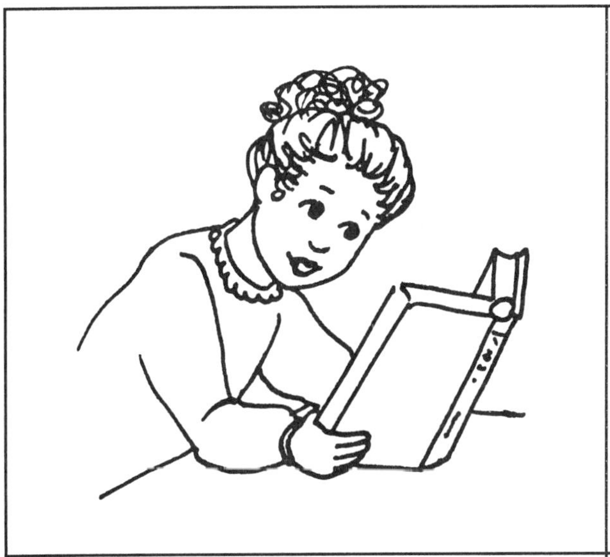
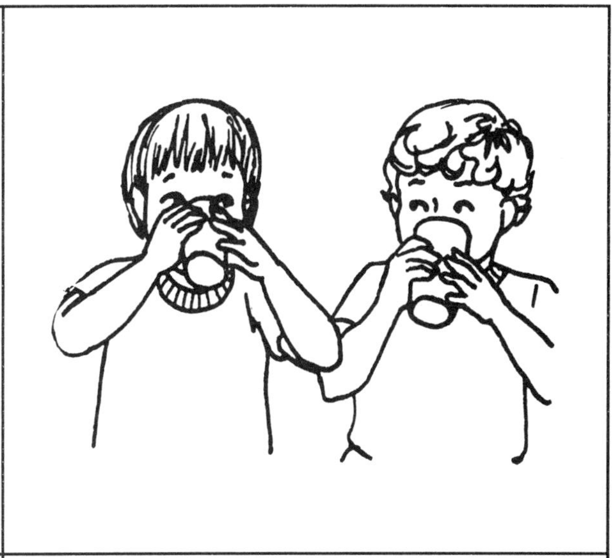
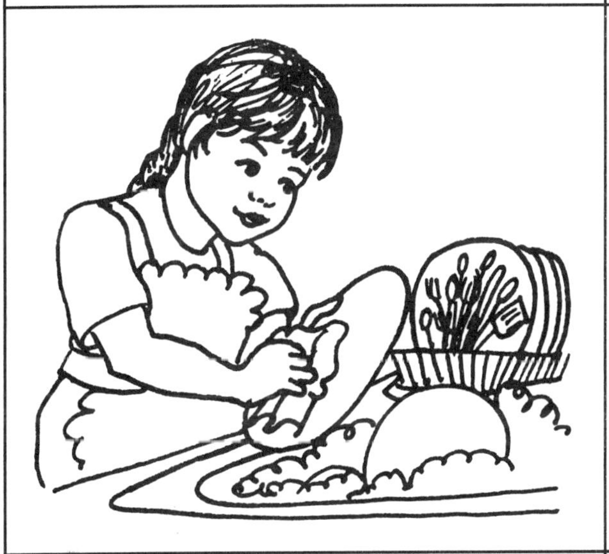
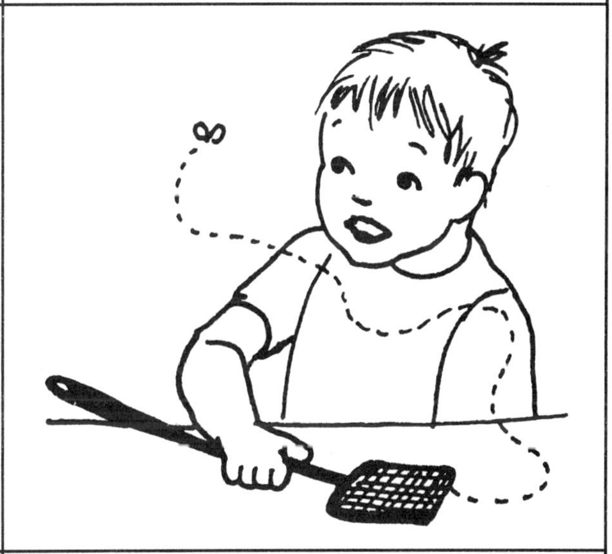
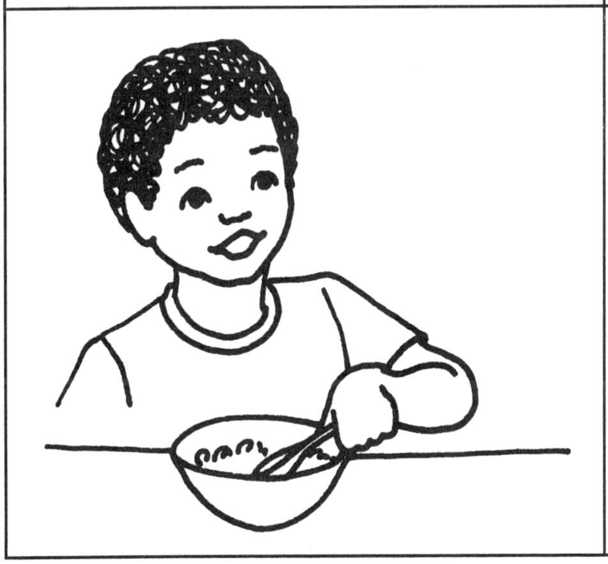
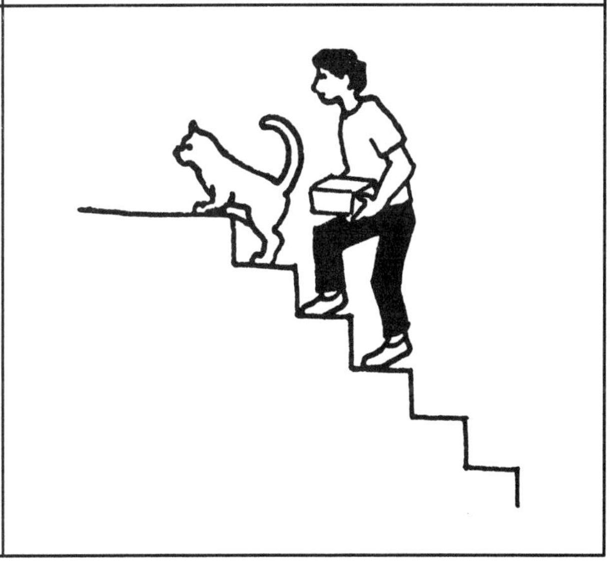

Materials: Pictures showing actions

6. *Show children action picture, such as boy eating cereal (page 97). Tell a story about the picture.*

A little boy woke up early one morning. The little boy went into the kitchen and saw his father fixing breakfast. The boy's father gave him a bowl of cereal. The little boy ate all the cereal because he was hungry.

Ask each child "Who," "What," "When," "Where," and "Why" questions.

Who is the story about? **When** did the boy get up? **Where** did the boy go when he got up? **Why** did he go into the kitchen? **Whom** did the boy see? **What** was the boy's father doing? **What** did the father give the boy? **Why** did the boy eat all the cereal?

Encourage use of complete sentences. Repeat activity, featuring other familiar stories.

PROGRESS CHECK

Materials: Pictures showing action

Show child action picture. Ask child "Who," "What," "When," "Where," and "Why" questions. Listen.

Scoring:

+	Responds to five "wh-" questions in complete sentences
0	Fails to respond to five "wh-" questions in complete sentences

Intermediate: Level C

Activity 5: Following Directions

Objective: To follow a three-part direction in sequence

Materials: None

1. I have a story to share. Please help me with the story. Listen carefully to my story.

   Whenever you hear me say the word "up," please hold up your hands. Whenever you hear me say the word "down," put your hands down. Ready? You must listen carefully. This is my story.

   As you tell the story, emphasize the words "up" and "down."

   A little girl named Sonja got up one morning. She went down the stairs to get her breakfast. After breakfast, she picked up her jacket and ran outside to play. She played for a long time. Then she decided to rest, so she sat down on a park bench.

   But oh! Sonja sat on a big wad of chewing gum. She was stuck; she stayed down. She tried and tried to stand up, but she just stayed down.

   Finally, she saw her friend, Timmy, and called to him, "Please help me get up; I am stuck down on this chewing gum."

   Timmy pulled and pulled and pulled and finally, up she came, and they both fell on the ground.

   What a funny sight! They laughed and laughed, and then Timmy and Sonja got up and went home.

   Allow all the children to participate in telling the story by putting their hands up and down at the correct cues.

2. Let's play "Simon Says."

   Give children simple directions to perform. Start with one-part directions. Then, give two-part directions. (Recommendation: If a child has difficulty remembering, have the child repeat the direction verbally before attempting to follow the direction.)

Materials:	Small table	Small chair
	Plastic bowl	Spoon
	Glass	Comb
	Hairbrush	Toothbrush
	Small mirror	Shirt

3. Let's talk about what we do to get ready for school.

Allow children to discuss their daily activities (such as washing hands and face, dressing, combing and brushing hair, and eating breakfast).

Now, let's pretend we are getting up and getting ready for school.

Give each child two-part directions to dramatize with props, such as:

____________________, wash your hands, then brush your hair.

____________________, put on your shirt, then eat your breakfast.

Give each child the opportunity to follow several two-part directions using props.

Materials: Classroom items

4. Let's play a game called "Can you find it?" I am going to ask each of you to find three objects and bring them here. Ready?

____________________, bring me a book, pencil, and piece of paper.

____________________, bring me a piece of chalk, a crayon, and a paintbrush.

Give each child an opportunity to participate. After all items have been brought, ask children to identify them.

5. *Display five objects. Review the names of those objects.*

We are going to play a game called "Stop." I am going to point to each object and say its name. Be careful. I might trick you and say the wrong name. I want you to listen carefully. If I say the wrong name, you say, "Stop." Ready? Listen carefully.

Tell names of objects, naming one or two objects incorrectly.

Repeat game several times.

6. I have a poem to share. *Teach.*

> Jeremiah blew the fire –
> Puff, puff, puff *(blow).*
> First, he blew it gently *(puff gently),*
> Then, he blew it rough *(blow hard).*

7. I have a story to share. Please help me with the story. Listen carefully to my story. I want you to do whatever I say in the story. Remember, you must listen carefully for my directions.

Tell story, using the names of children in the group in the story. This is my story:

> Once there were four children named Meredith, Jeremy, Joseph, and Sandy. They woke up on bright morning, rubbed their eyes *(rub eyes),* and stretched *(stretch).* Then, they washed their faces *(wash face)* and put on their school clothes *(dress).*
>
> When they were dressed, they went to the kitchen to eat a bowl of cereal for breakfast *(eat cereal).*
>
> Before leaving for school, the children brushed their teeth *(brush teeth),* they combed their hair *(comb hair),* and put on their coats *(put on coats).* It was such a pretty day, they decided to walk to school *(stamp feet).*
>
> When they saw the school ahead of them, they were so excited that they ran to the front door *(stamp feet quickly).* They tried to open the front door *(open door),* but it was locked!
>
> They looked around *(look around).* They saw no other children. Oh no! It was Saturday!

Materials: Paper stars (page 92)
Tape

8. *Put a piece of rolled tape on back of each star so it can stick to other objects; give each child one.*

We are going to play "Follow The Leader." We will use these stars.

Listen carefully, and the leader will tell you what to do with your star. I will be the leader first. Ready?

> Stick your star on your knee. Good.
> Now, stick your star on your chin. Good.
> Stick your star on the table. *Continue giving directions to be followed.*

Now, you take turns being the leader. Remember, the leader will tell us what to do with our stars. ____________________, you go first.

Now, when we play the game, I will give you three directions to follow, so listen carefully to my directions. Ready?

Put the star on your foot, raise your hand, and stand up. Good.
Stick the star on your nose, clap your hands, and put it on the table.

9. I have a poem to share. *Teach "The Grand Old Duke of York:"*

Oh, the Grand Old Duke of York,
He had ten thousand men.
He marched them up the hill *(stand up)*
And marched them down again *(sit down).*

And when they're up, they're up *(stand up),*
And when they're down, they're down *(sit down).*
And when they're only halfway up *(stand partially),*
They're neither up *(stand)* nor down *(sit).*

Materials: Tissue Tape

10. *Place a piece of rolled tape on back of each tissue so it can stick to other objects. Give each child a tissue.*

We're going to play "Follow The Leader." We'll use these tissues. Listen carefully, and the leader will tell you what to do with your tissue. I will be the leader first. Ready?

Stick your tissue on your knee. Good.
Now, stick your tissue on your chin. Good. Stick it on the table.

Continue giving directions to be followed. Praise all actions.

Now, you take turns being the leader. Remember, the leader will tell us what to do with our tissues. ____________________, you go first.

Now, when we play the game, I will give you three directions to follow, so listen carefully to my directions. Ready?

Put the tissue on your foot, raise your hand, and stand up. Good.
Stick the tissue on your nose, clap your hands, and put it on the table.

Continue giving three-part directions. Praise all actions.

Materials: Paper stars Tape Tissues

11. *Place a piece of rolled tape on back of each star so it can stick to other objects.*

    We are going to play "Follow the Leader." We will use these stars and these tissues. *Give each child star and tissue.*

    Listen carefully and the leader will tell you what to do with your star and your tissues. I will be the leader first. Ready?

    Stick your star on your knee and the tissue on the table. Good.

    Now, stick your star on your chin and your tissue in your lap. Good.

    Continue giving directions to be followed. Praise. Allow each child to go individually.

    Now, you take turns being the leaders. Remember, the leader must tell us what to do with our stars and tissue. ____________________, you go first.

    Now, when we play the game, I will give you three directions to follow, so listen carefully to all three of my directions. Ready?

    Put the star on your foot, the tissue on your head, and stand up. Good. Stick the star on your nose, put the tissue on the table, and clap your hands.

    Continue giving three-part directions.

12. I am going to ask each of you to do two things. Listen carefully and remember both things. Ready?

    Give children in turn two-part directions to complete (give errands in room or ask them to dramatize actions).

    ____________________, please get an eraser and put it on my desk.
    Continue giving each child an opportunity to participate.

    Now, I am going to ask you to do three things. Listen carefully and remember all three things. Ready?

    Give children in turn three-part directions to follow.

13. *Read a poem that includes gestures, such as "Mr. Tall and Mr. Small" by Beatrice Wells Carson.*

PROGRESS CHECK

Materials:	Pencil	Crayon
	Book	Ball

Materials: Common objects (such as eraser, chalk, book)

Listen carefully. I am going to ask you to do three things.

> Please get an eraser, put it on my desk, and close the door. Good.
> Now, pick up the chalk, mark on the board, and sit down. *Observe.*

Scoring:

+	Follows three-part direction in sequence without any prompts
0	Fails to follow three-part direction in sequence without any prompts

Intermediate: Level D

Activity 1: Categories

Objective: To classify objects in categories

Materials: Four articles of clothing; Four items that are not clothing; Four toys; Box; Large bag

1. We are going to talk about clothes; clothes are what we wear. Look at my clothes. *Name items being worn, and point to each one.* I am wearing a dress and a pair of shoes. Because it is cold today, I wore a coat and gloves to school. Now, let's look at the clothes you are wearing. *Ask each child to name articles of clothing.*

   Display all items and the bag. Let's play "Bag It." Here's how to play:

   > Choose an item from the pile. If the item is something to wear, put the item in our clothes bag. *Point to bag.* If the item is not something to wear, put the item over here. *Indicate a place.* Ready? *Allow each child to select an item; group accordingly.*
   >
   > Let's look at the items we put in our clothes bag. *Remove items from the bag, and ask the children to name each one.*
   >
   > Let's see how many kinds of clothes we can name. I will count them. *As the children name the items, count aloud. Praise responses and actions.*

2. We are going to talk about toys. Toys are what we play with. Look around the room. Tell what toys you see. *Allow each child to respond.* What are your favorite toys? *Ask each child individually.*

   Display all items. Let's play "Bag It." Here's how to play:

   > Choose an item from this pile. If it is something to wear, put it in our clothes bag. *Point to the bag.* If the item is a toy, put it in the toy box. *Point to the box.* Ready? *Allow each child to do the activity.*
   >
   > Let's look at the items we put in our clothes bag. *Remove items from the bag, and ask the children to name each item. Repeat procedure for the toys in the box.*
   >
   > Let's see how many toys we can name. I'll count. *As children name toys, count aloud.*

Materials: Four items of clothing
Four toys
Four foods
Three large bags (one with a picture of a sock taped on it, one with a picture of a cake taped on it, and one with a picture of a toy taped on it)

3. We are going to talk about foods. Food is what we eat. What are your favorite foods? *Allow each child the opportunity to respond.*

   Display items. Let's play "Bag It." Here's how to play:

   > Pick an item from this pile. If the item is something to wear, put the item in our clothes bag. *Point to the bag with the sock.* If the item is a toy, put the item in the toy bag. *Point to the bag with the toy.* If the item is something to eat, put the item in the food bag. *Point to the bag with the cake.* Ready? *Ask each child to select an item; group accordingly.*
   >
   > Let's look at the items we put in our clothes bag. *Remove items from bag, and ask the children to name each one. Repeat procedures for toys and foods.*
   >
   > Let's see how many foods we can name. I will keep count. *As children name foods, count them aloud.*

   I am going to name three things. I want you to tell if they are clothes, foods, or toys. For example, if I say "shirt," "shoe," and "sock," you say, "They are all clothes." Ready? *Allow each child to name three items from a category.*

Materials: Eight items of clothing
Eight toys
Eight foods
Three large bags (one with a picture of a sock taped on it, one with a picture of a cake taped on it, and one with a picture of a toy taped on it)

4. *Display all items.* Let's play "Bag It." Choose something from this pile.

   > If it is something to wear, put it in the clothes bag. *Point to bag with sock.*
   > If it is something to play with, put it in the toy bag. *Point to bag with toy.*
   > If it is something to eat, put it in the food bag. *Point to bag with cake.*

   Let's look at what we put in the clothes bag. *Remove items from bag; ask children to name each one. Repeat with toys and foods.*

   Now, I am going to name three things. Tell me if they are all clothes, all foods, or all toys. For example, if I name "shirt," "shoe," and "sock," you will say, "They are all clothes." Ready? *Allow each child to tell the category for three items.*

People

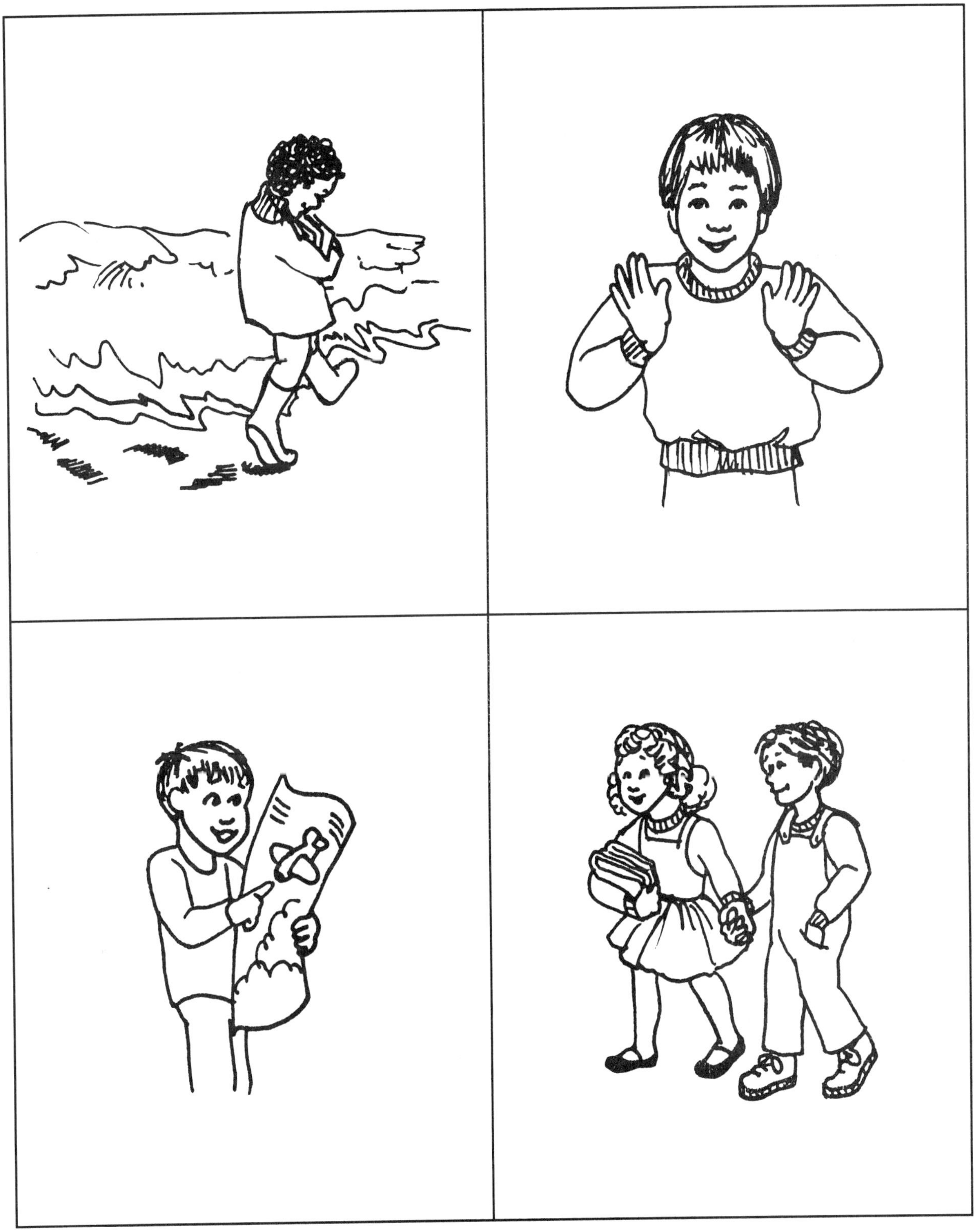

Transportation

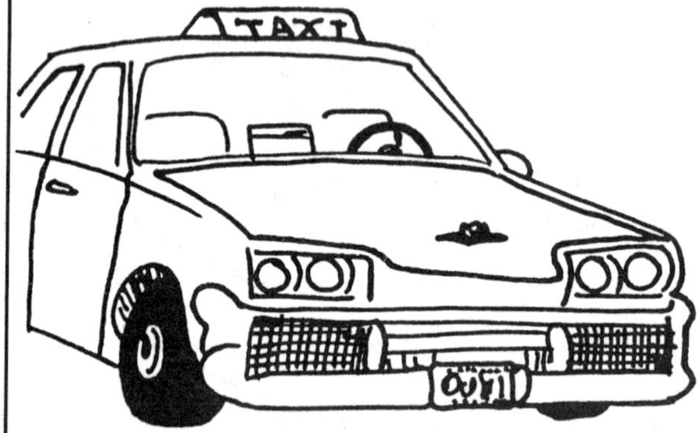

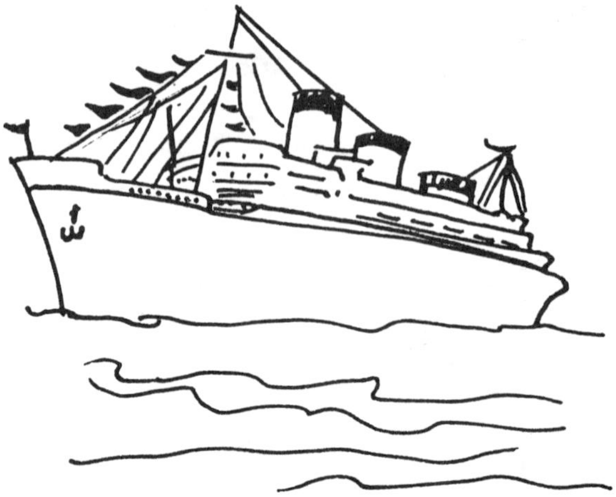

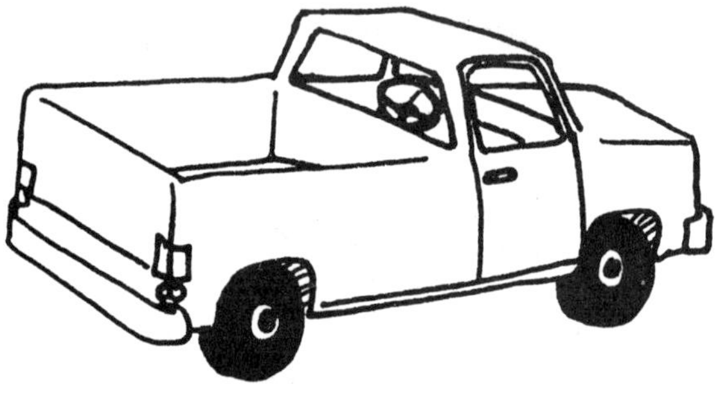

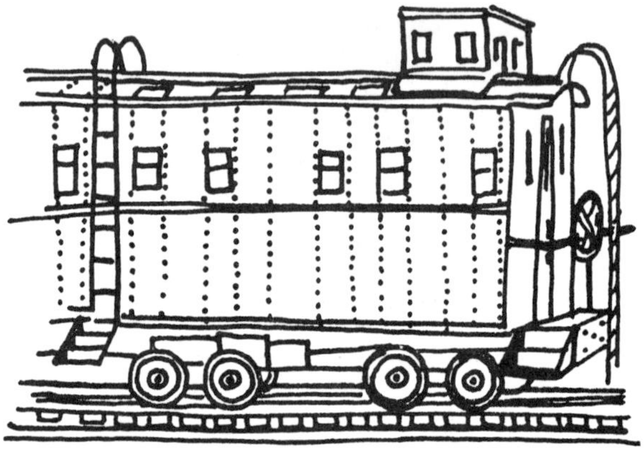

Furniture

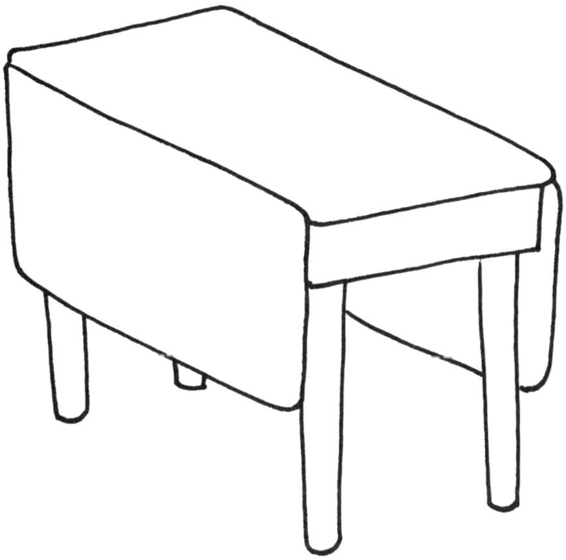

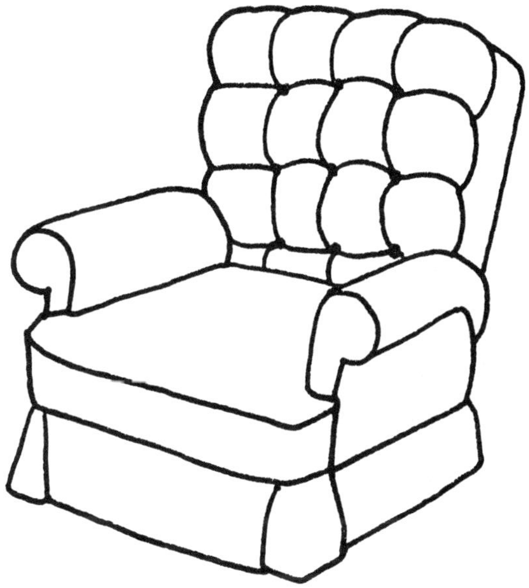

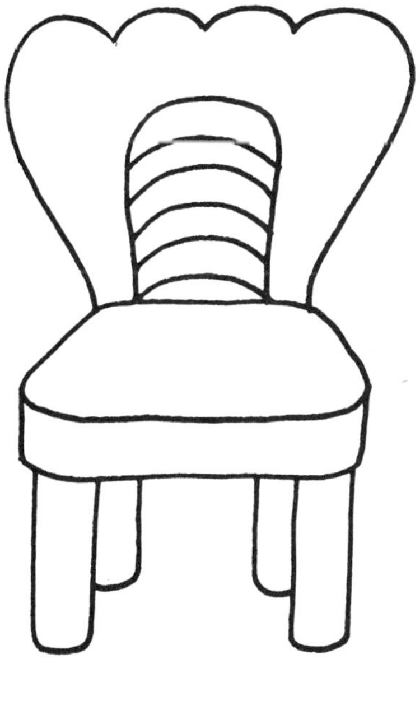

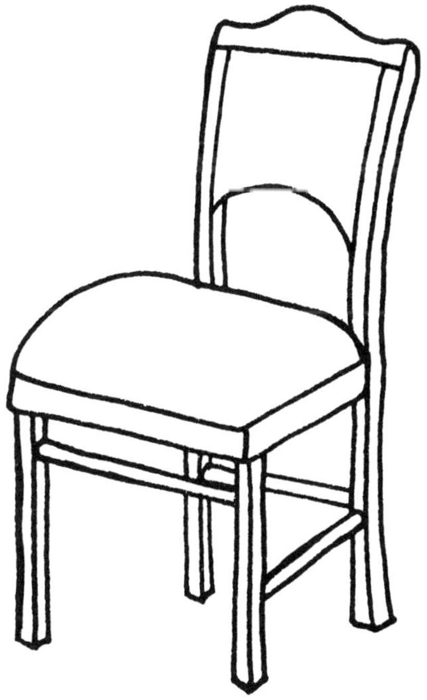

Animals

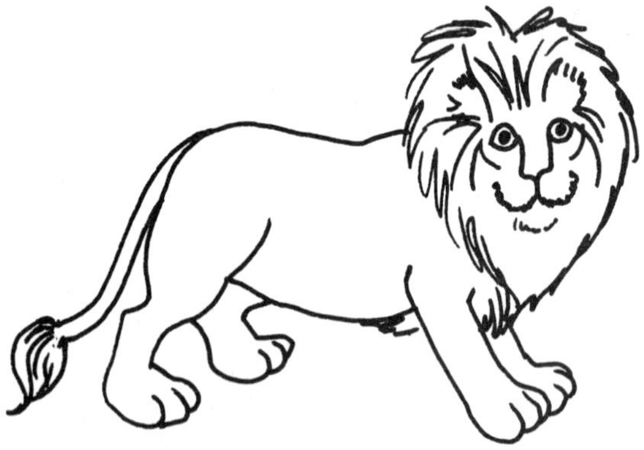

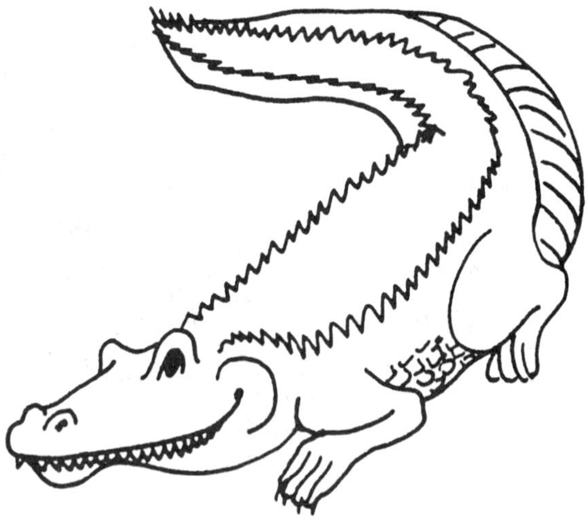

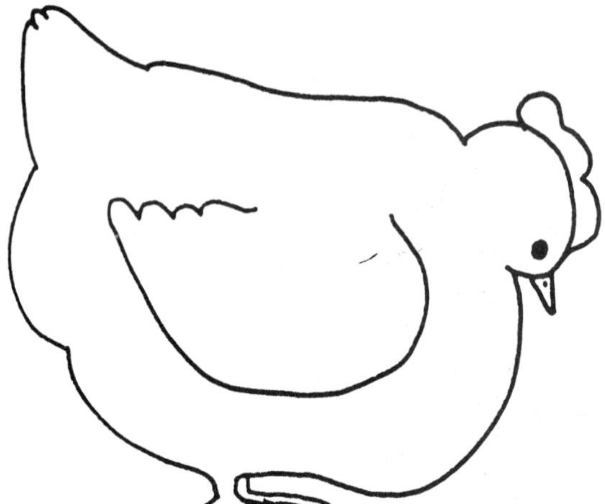

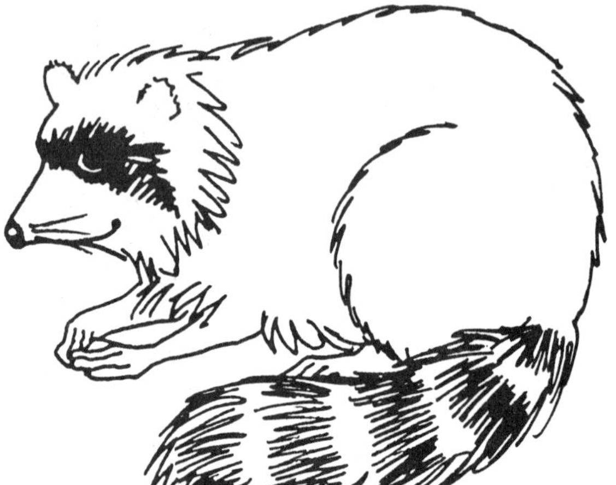

Plants

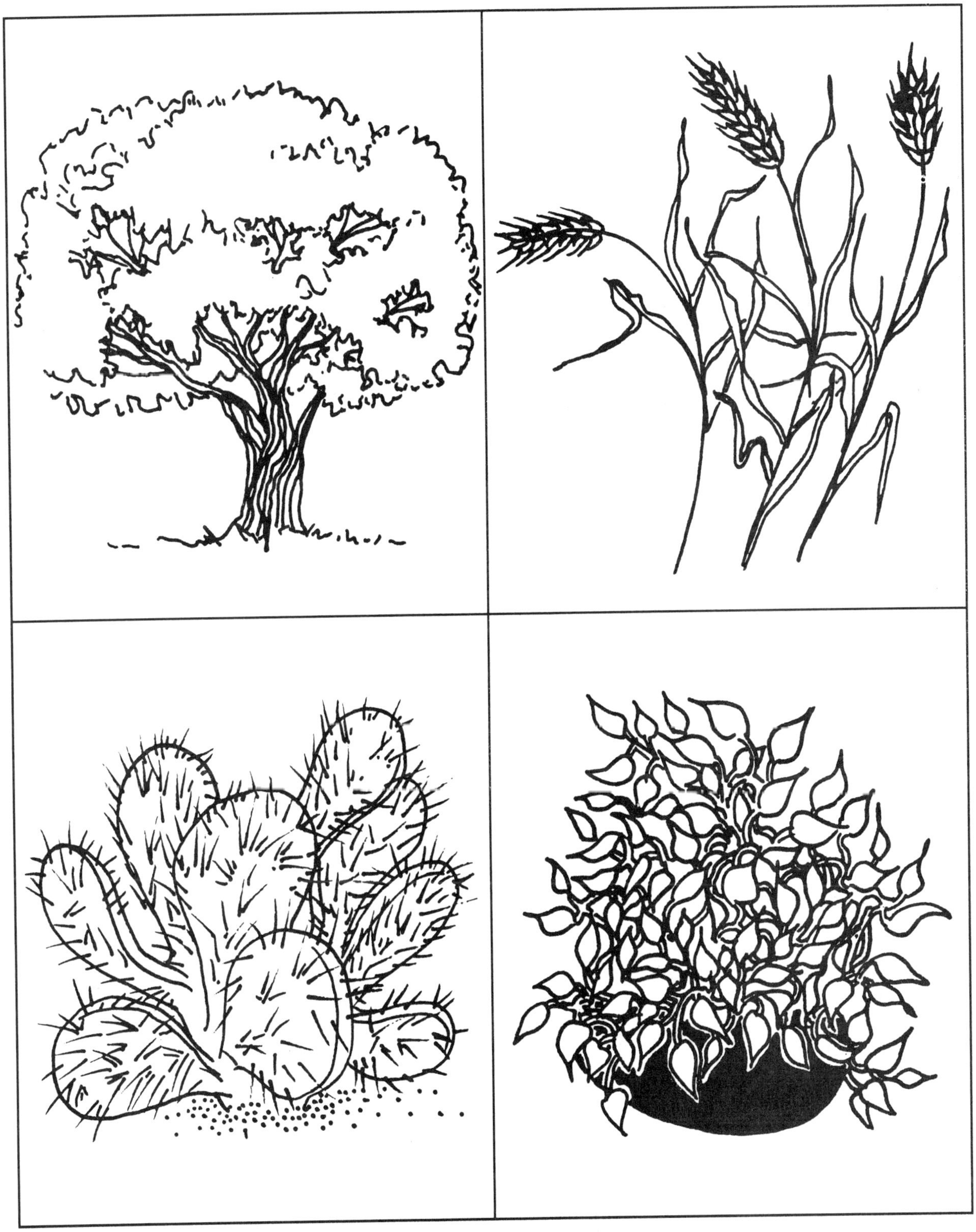

Body Parts

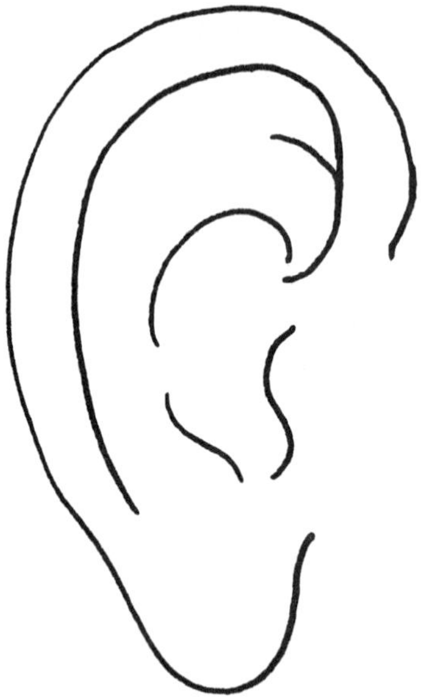

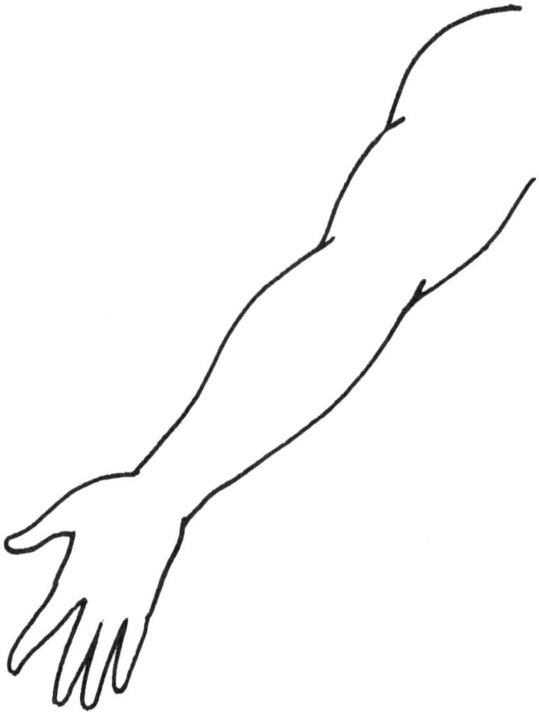

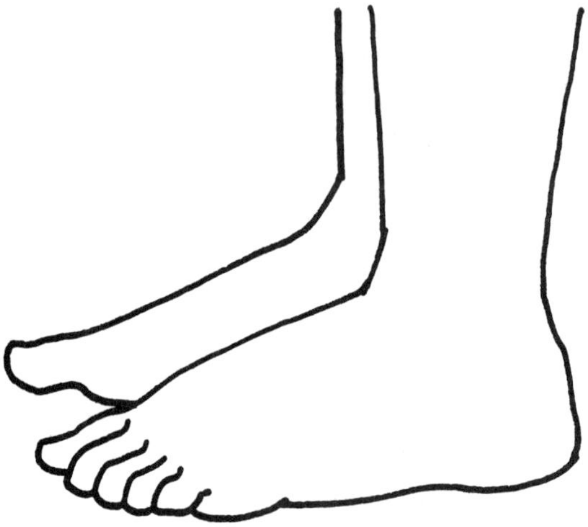

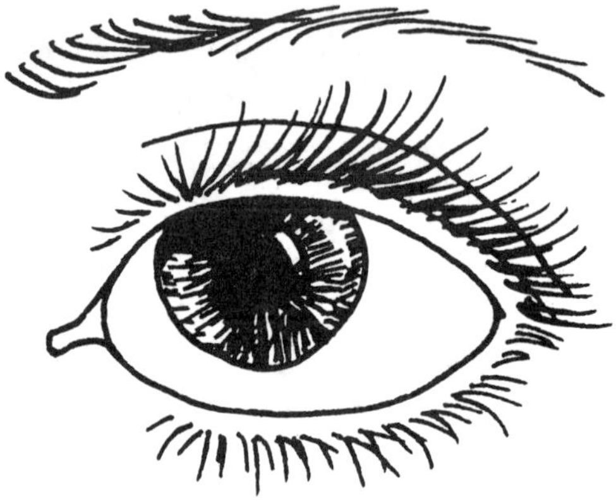

Materials: Four pictures of people
Four pictures of kinds of transportation

5. *Show children pictures of people.* These are pictures of people. We are all people. *Present each picture; discuss its content.* Who are some of your favorite people?

   Show children pictures of transportation. These are pictures of kinds of transportation, things we can ride.

   Present each picture; discuss its content. What kinds of transportation have you ridden?

   > I am going to mix up the pictures of people and transportation, then put them on the table so you can see them. *Display pictures.* Choose a picture that shows people, and put it here. *Indicate place. Allow each child to participate individually.* Now, pick a picture that shows transportation, and put it over there. *Indicate place. Ask each child individually.*

   Point to pictures of people. Say: All these pictures are pictures of people. *Review each picture with the children.*

   Repeat procedure with Transportation pictures.

Materials: Four pictures of animals
Four pictures of plants

6. *Show children pictures of animals.* These are pictures of animals. *Present each picture; discuss its content.* What are your favorite animals?

   Show children pictures of plants. These are pictures of plants. *Present each picture; discuss its content.* What kinds of plants are in your yard? *If possible, go to a window or outside doorway.* What plants do you see outside?

   > I am going to mix up the pictures of animals and plants. I will put them on the table so you can see them. *Display pictures.* Choose a picture that is an animal, and put the picture of the animal here. *Indicate place. Allow each child to respond.* Now, pick a picture that is a plant, and put the picture of the plant over there *(indicate a place). Ask each child individually. Point to animal pictures.* All these pictures are pictures of animals. *Review each picture with the children. Repeat procedure with pictures of plants.*

Materials: Four pictures of furniture
Four pictures of body parts

7. *Show children pictures of furniture.* These are pictures of furniture. We have furniture in this room and in our houses. *Present each picture; discuss its content.* What furniture do you see in this room? *Praise.*

   Show children pictures of body parts. These are pictures of parts of our bodies. *Present each picture; discuss its content.* What other body parts do we have?

   I'm going to mix up the pictures of furniture and the pictures of body parts and put them on the table so you can see them. *Display pictures.* Pick a picture that shows furniture, and put the picture here. *Indicate place. Allow each child to answer individually.* Now, pick a picture that is a part of our body, and put the picture over there. *Indicate place. Ask each child to respond.*

Materials: Four pictures each of:

People	Kinds of transportation
Animals	Plants
Furniture	Body parts

8. *Display pictures.* Let's play "Name and Sort." Here's how to play:

   Hold up picture of people. This picture shows people. I will put it here. *Indicate place.*

   Continue procedure, displaying one picture from each category (transportation, animals, plants, people, furniture, body parts) and indicating its position. Place remaining pictures in a stack.

   Take a picture from the top of the pile. Show the picture and tell if it shows people, transportation, animals, plants, furniture, or parts of the body. Then, put the picture in the correct place. Ready?

PROGRESS CHECK

Materials: Four pictures each of:

People	Kinds of transportation
Animals	Plants
Furniture	Body parts

Display pictures. Ask the child to select a picture, identify the category, and select two other pictures that belong to that category. Ask the child follow this procedure for all categories.

Scoring:

+	Names the categories and sorts correctly
0	Fails to name the categories and sort correctly

Intermediate: Level D

Activity 2: Quantitative Concepts

Objective: To name quantitative concepts

BIG and LITTLE

Materials: Four pairs of objects, each pair similar except for size (such as big and little scissors, blocks, pieces of paper)
Pictures of big and little animals and objects

1. *Display objects. Introduce concepts of "big" and "little." Hold up big scissors.* This is a big pair of scissors. *Hold up child's scissors.* This is a little pair of scissors. *Continue procedure with other objects. Scramble objects.* Let's play "Name and Sort."

   Hold up big scissors. Are these scissors big or little? Yes, they are big. We are going to put all the big items here. *Indicate place. Hold up child's scissors.* What size are these scissors? Yes, they are little. We are going to put the little items over there. *Indicate place.* Choose an object, tell if it is big or little, and put it in the correct place. *Ask each child to answer.*

   Display pictures. These pictures are of items that are big or little. *Show pictures of an ant and an elephant.* Which picture is big? Yes, the elephant is big. Which picture is little? Yes, the ant is little. *Continue procedure for other pictures.*

   When finished: Let's play "Name and Sort." *Hold up picture of elephant.* Is this elephant big or little? Yes, the elephant is big. We are going to put all the big items here. *Indicate place. Hold up picture of an ant.* What size is this ant? Yes, the ant is little. We are going to put the little items over there. *Indicate place.* Choose a picture. Tell if the object in the picture is big or little, and put it in the correct place. *Allow each child to answer individually.*

LONG and SHORT

Materials: Four pairs of objects, each pair similar except for length (long and short strips of paper, pieces of yarn, straws, pencils)
Pairs of pictures of short and long objects

2. *Display objects. Introduce concepts of "short" and "long." Hold up a long strip of paper.* This is a long piece of paper. *Hold up a short piece of paper.* This is a short piece of paper. *Continue procedure with other objects. Scramble objects.* Let's play "Name and Sort."

Hold up a long strip of paper. Is this paper short or long? Yes, this paper is long. We are going to put all the long items here. *Indicate place. Select an object, tell if it is short or long, and put it in the correct place. Ask each child to respond.*

> *Display pictures.* These pictures are of things that are short or long. *Show pictures of girls who have short and long hair.* Which picture shows something short? Yes, this girl has short hair. *Continue procedure for other pictures. When finished:* Let's play "Name and Sort."

Hold up picture of short hair. Is this hair short or long? Yes, the hair is short. We are going to put all the short items here. *Indicate place. Hold up picture of girl with long hair.* Is the girl's hair short or long? Yes, the girl's hair is long. We are going to put the long items over there. *Indicate place.* Choose a picture. Tell if the object in the picture is short or long, and put it in the correct place. *Allow each child to respond.*

HEAVY and LIGHT

Materials: Four pairs of objects, each pair similar except for weight (heavy and light balls, blocks, toys, plastic eggs)
Pairs of pictures of heavy and light objects

3. *Display objects. Introduce concepts of "heavy" and "light." Hold up a baseball.* This is a heavy ball. *Hold up a sponge ball.* This is a light ball. *Continue procedure with other objects. Scramble objects.* Let's play "Name and Sort."

Hold up baseball. Is this baseball heavy or light? Yes, the baseball is heavy. We are going to put all the heavy items here. *Indicate place. Hold up sponge ball.* Is this ball heavy or light? Yes, this ball is light. We are going to put the light items over there. *Indicate place.* Choose an object, tell if it is heavy or light, and put it in the correct place. *Ask each child individually.*

> *Display pictures.* These pictures are of items that are heavy and light. *Show pictures of ball and balloon.* Which picture shows something heavy? Yes, this ball is heavy. Which picture shows something light? Yes, this balloon is light. *Continue procedure for other pictures. When finished:* Let's play "Name and Sort."

Hold up picture of baseball. Is this ball heavy or light? Yes, the ball is heavy. We are going to put all the heavy items here. *Indicate place. Hold up picture of balloon.* Is this heavy or light? Yes, this is light. We are going to put the light items over there. *Indicate place.* Pick a picture. Tell if the picture is of something heavy or light, and put the picture in the correct place. *Allow each child to respond individually.*

Big and Little Objects

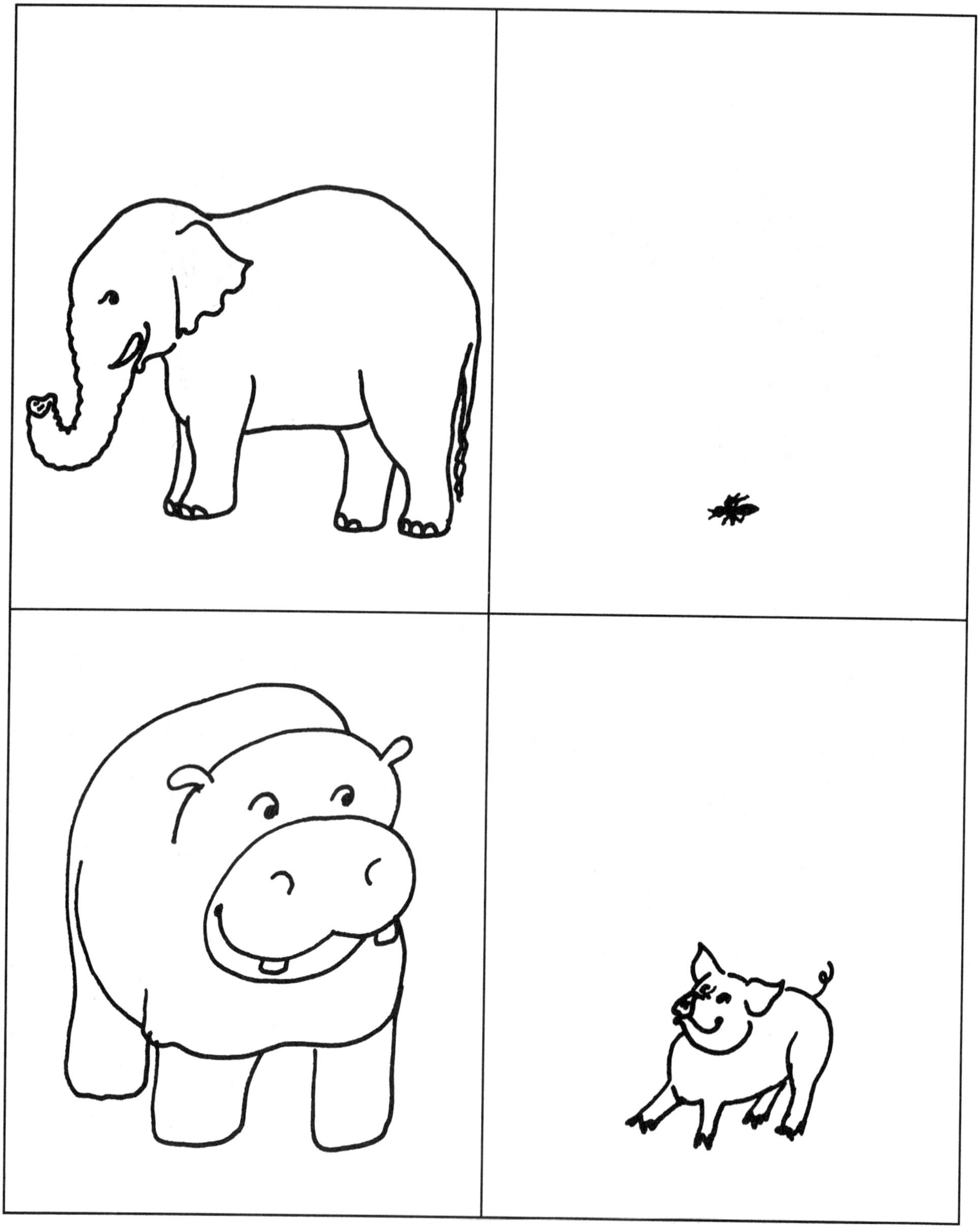

Long and Short Objects

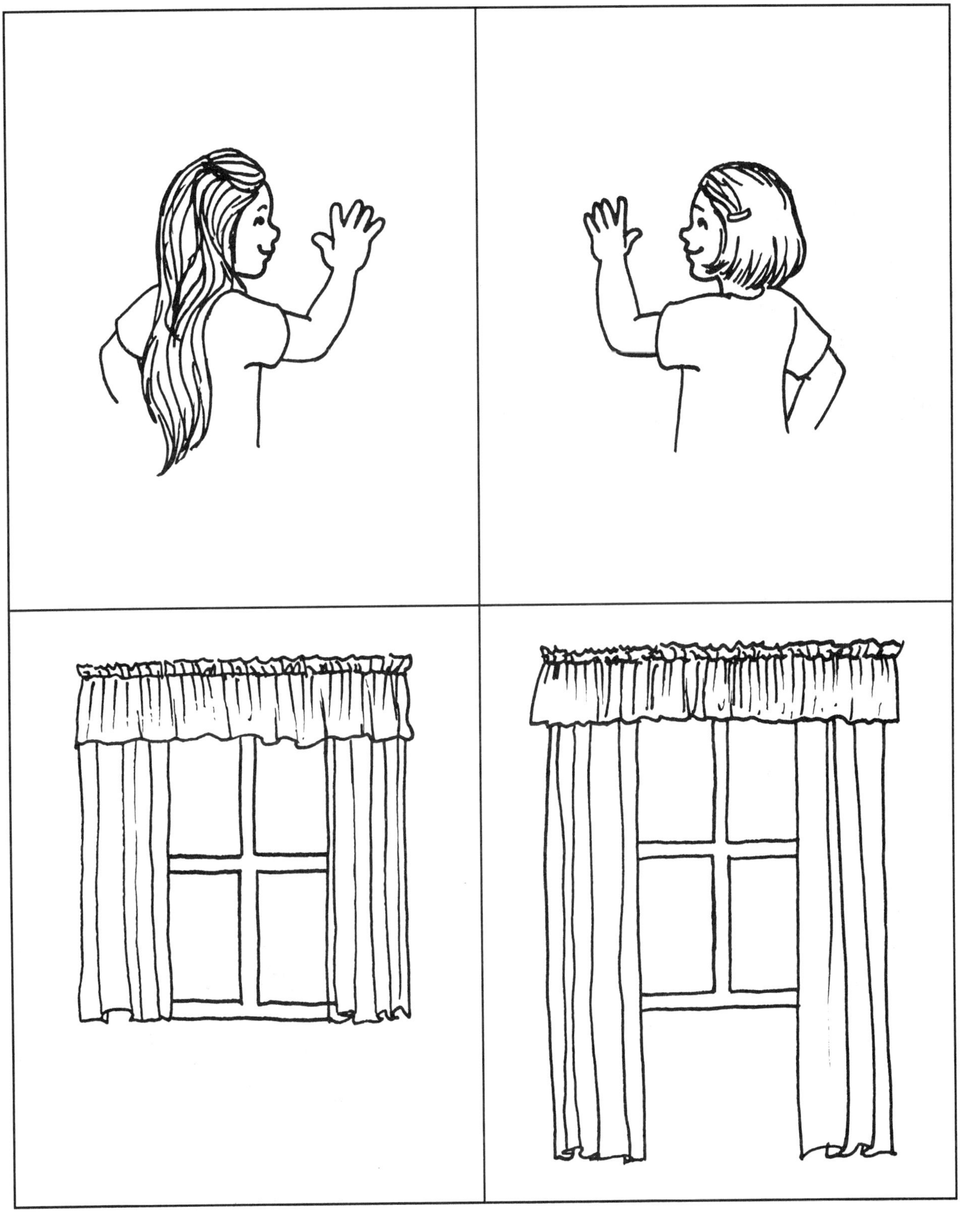

Heavy and Light Objects

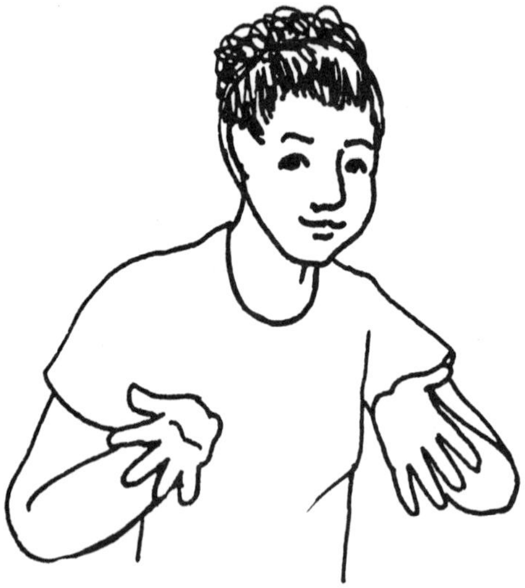

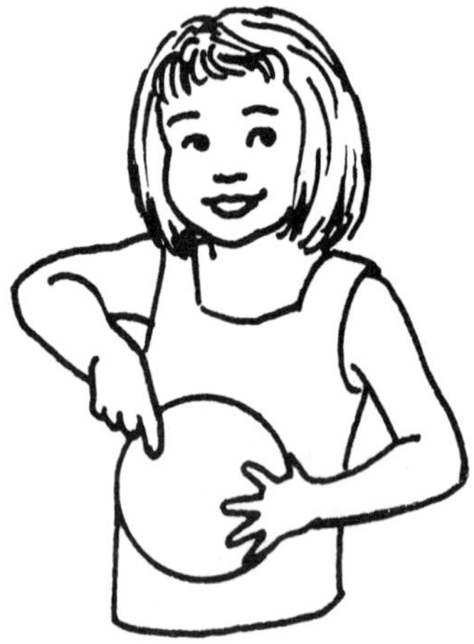

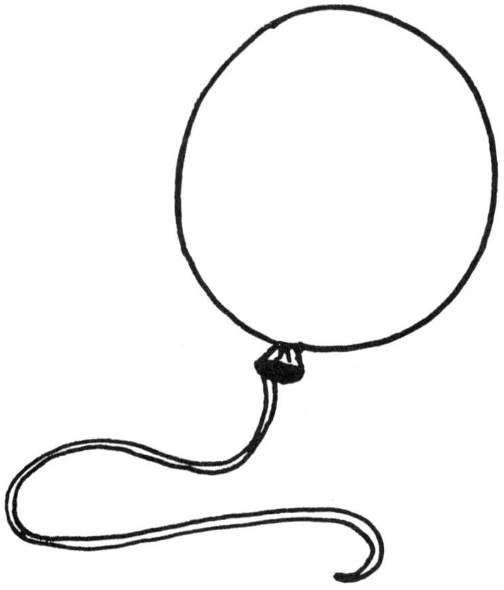

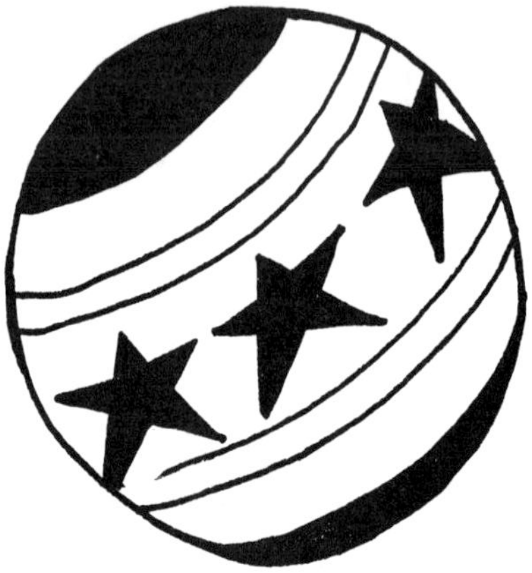

Tall and Short Objects

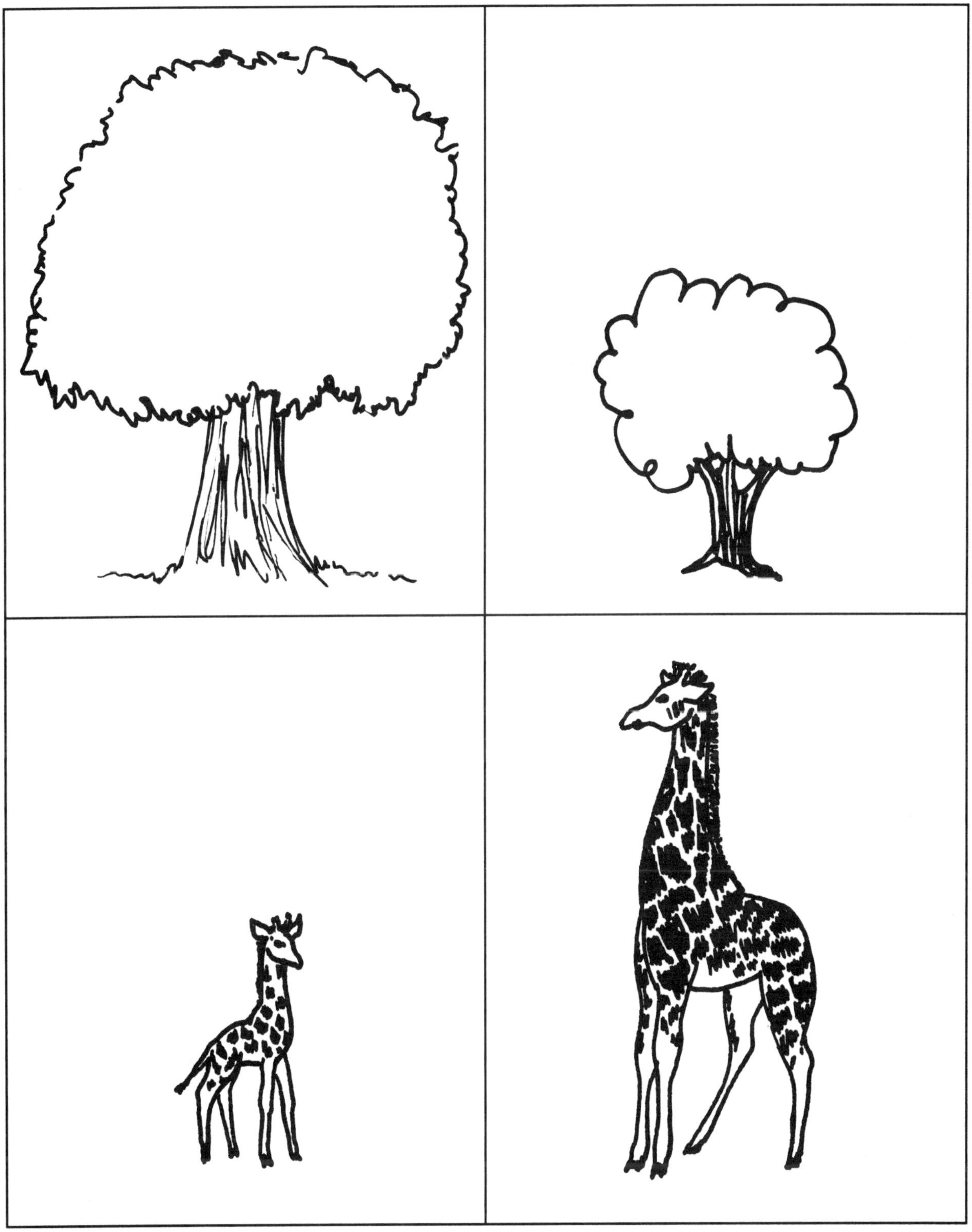

TALL and SHORT

Materials: Blocks to make a tall stack and a short stack
Large bag
Pairs of pictures of:
- Tall and short objects
- Heavy and light objects
- Long and short objects
- Big and little objects

4. *Introduce concepts of "tall" and "short." Ask a child to stand beside you.*

> ___________________, please stand beside me. Everyone, look at the two of us. I am tall, and ___________________ is short. "Tall" and "short" are opposites.
>
> Let's practice tall and short. I want all of you to make yourselves as tall as you can. Stand on your tiptoes, and stretch your arms up high. Now try to make yourselves as short as you can by squatting down.

Display blocks. Make a tall stack and a short stack. Point to the short stack. Is this stack short or tall? Yes, this stack is short. *Point to tall stack; ask children if this stack is short or tall. Allow each child to respond as you point to a stack.*

Display pictures. These pictures are of things that are short or tall. *Show picture of short and tall people,* Which picture shows something short? Yes, this is a picture of a short person. Which picture shows something tall. Yes, this picture shows a tall person.

Continue procedure for other pictures. When finished: You choose a picture, and tell if the picture is short or tall. *Ask each child.*

Review opposites introduced previously ("light" and "heavy," "big" and "little," and "short" and "long," using pictures or objects).

Thick and Thin, Full and Empty, Many and Few

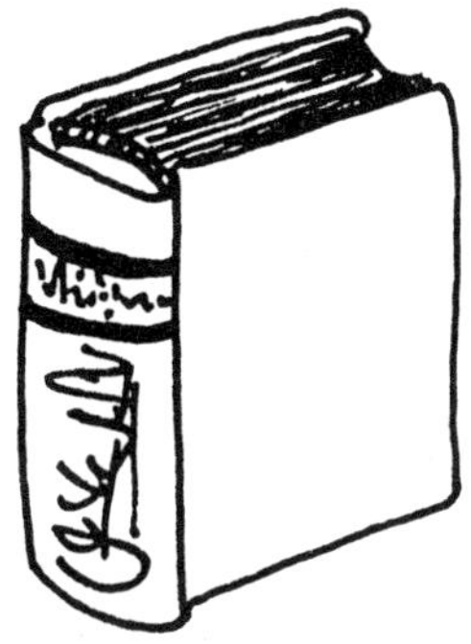

thick

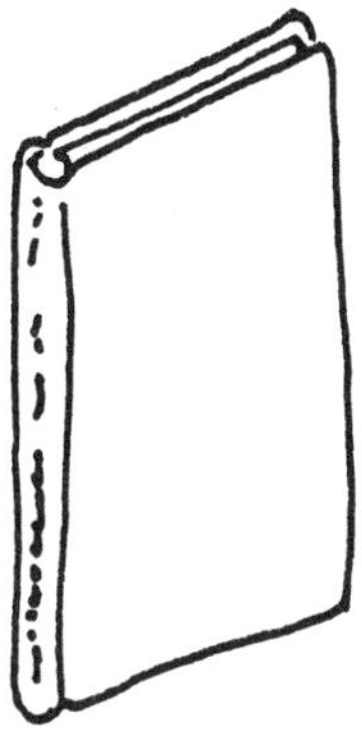

thin

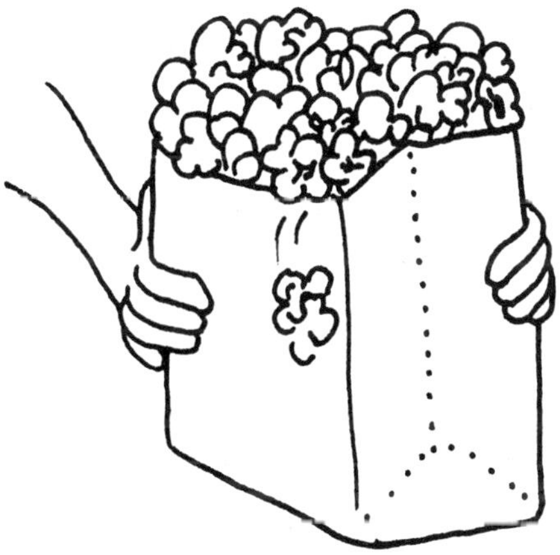

full

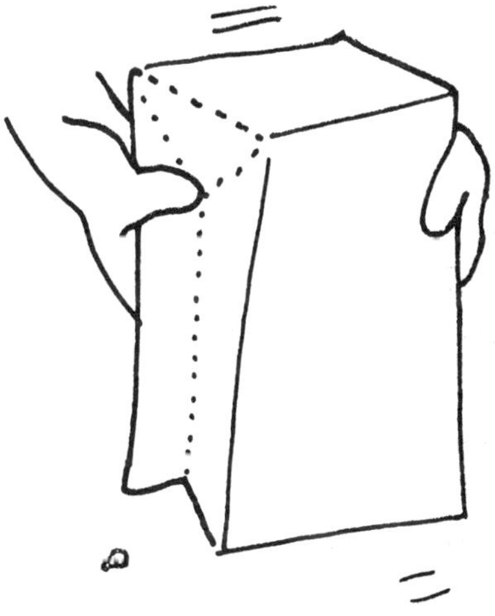

empty

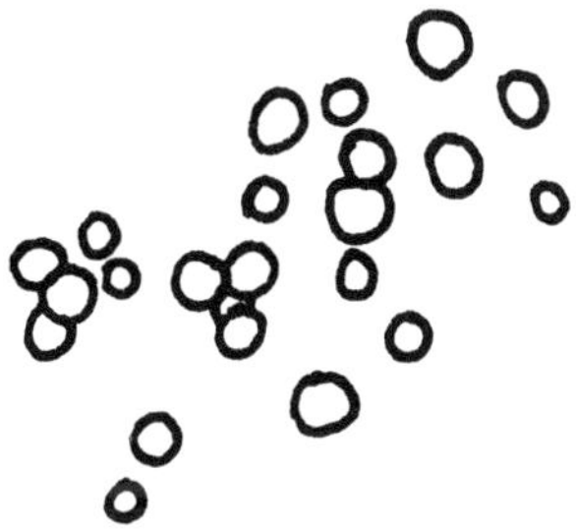

many

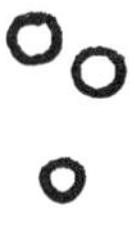

few

FULL and EMPTY

Materials: Two glasses or cups
Pictures or container of water
Ten small containers (five full and five empty)

5. *Introduce concepts "full" and "empty." Display pitcher and two glasses. Point to glasses.* These glasses do not have anything in them. They are empty. I can turn the glasses upside down, and nothing comes out. *Demonstrate.*

   Hold up one glass. I am going to fill this glass with water. *Pour water into glass to top.* This glass is filled to the top with water. This glass is full. I cannot put any more water in this glass. If I do, the water will spill over. *Point to empty glass.* This glass is empty. *Point to full glass.* This glass is full. I will point to a glass. You decide if the glass is full or empty. Say "the glass is full," or "the glass is empty." Ready? *Point to glasses; ask each child to respond.*

   Display containers. Scramble positions of full and empty ones. Look at these containers. Some of them are full. *Point to a full container.* Let's put the full containers over here. *Move full container to place.* Some of the containers are empty. *Point to empty container.* Let's put the empty containers here. *Move empty container to place.* Choose a container, and tell if it is full or empty. Say "this is full" or "this is empty." Then, put the container in the correct place. Ready? *Ask each child to pick container, identify, and place.*

MORE and LESS

Materials: Snacks (cereal, raisins, bread cubes, grapes)
Napkins or paper towels
Twelve cards (six each with two large dots, six each with five large dots)

6. *Introduce concepts of "more" and "less."* Let's stand up. *Divide children into two unequal (by at least two children) groups.* Now, we have two groups. Which group has more children? Yes, this group has more *(point).* Which group has less children? Yes, this group has less *(point).* We can say groups have more children *(point)* or less children *(point).*

   Put snacks on table and two napkins in the center. Put one piece of snack on a napkin and a handful of snacks on the other napkin. Which napkin has more? Yes, this napkin has more *(point).* Which napkin has less? Yes, *(point)* this napkin has less. *Give each child two napkins or paper towels. Put one piece of snack on napkin. Put a handful of snacks on the other napkin.* Look at your napkins. Point to the napkin that has more. Yes, the napkin with a handful of snacks has more. Which napkin has less? Yes, the napkin with only one piece has less.

Display cards. Scramble and divide cards into two piles. Let's play a card game called "More or Less." *Ask two children at a time to draw a card.* I'll ask two people to take a card from each pile. The person who has the card with "more" on it gets to keep both cards. __________________ and __________________, please draw a card. Who has the card with "more" on it? Yes, __________________ has the card with "more" on it; it does not have "few" on it. __________________ keeps the cards. *Continue play. If two children draw cards with same amount, return cards to bottom of pile and draw again.*

MANY and FEW

Materials: Twelve blocks
Twelve pencils or crayons
Twelve cards (two of each: two large dots, three large dots, four large dots, eight large dots, nine large dots, and ten large dots)

7. *Introduce the concepts of "many" and "few."* Let's stand up. *Divide children into two unequal groups.* Now, we have two groups. Which group has many children in it? Yes, this group *(point)* has many children. Which group has few children? Yes, this group *(point)* has few children. We can say our groups have many children *(point)* or few children *(point).*

    Display blocks with eight in one pile and four in another pile. Which pile has many blocks? Which pile has few blocks? *Allow each child to respond.*

    Display crayons or pencils with eight in one pile and four in another pile. Which pile has many crayons? Which pile has few crayons? *Allow each child to respond.*

    Display cards. Scramble cards, and divide them into two piles. Let's play a card game called "Many or Few." *Ask two children at a time to draw a card.* I will ask two people to draw a card from each pile. The person who has the card with "many" on it gets to keep both cards. __________________ and __________________, please draw a card. Who has the card with "many" on it? Yes, __________________ has the card with "many" on it and not have "few" on it. __________________ keeps the cards. *Continue play. If two children draw cards with same amount, return cards to bottom of piles and redraw.*

REVIEW

Materials: Pictures to demonstrate concepts of "full" and "empty," "more" and "less," and "few" and "many."

8. *Place "full" or "empty" pictures face down.* Choose a picture, and show it to us. Tell if the object in the picture is full or empty. Watch. *Show picture to group.* This is a (full *or* empty) __________________ *(name object). Continue procedure with other groups of pictures. Discuss and praise all responses.*

PROGRESS CHECK

Materials: Pairs of pictures of –
Tall and short objects
Heavy and light objects
Short and long objects
Big and little

1. *Display pictures or objects by category* ("big" and "little;" "long" and "short;" "heavy" and "light;" "tall" and "short"). *Select a picture or object from the "big" and "little" group and say:* "Tell if this picture is big or little." *Repeat procedure, selecting pictures or objects from each group.*

Scoring:

+	Correctly identifies all four concepts
0	Fails to identify all four concepts correctly

Materials: Pictures to demonstrate concepts of "full" and "empty," "more" and "less," and "many" and "few"

2. *Put pictures face down by category: full and empty; more and less; few and many.* Choose a picture from the first group; tell if the object it shows is full or empty. *Repeat this procedure with the remaining two groups.*

Scoring:

+	Identifies the pictures correctly
0	Fails to identify the pictures correctly

Intermediate: Level D

Activity 3: Sentences

Objective: To use complete sentences to answer questions

Materials: Common classroom objects

1. Let's play "Pretend." I will give each of you something to pretend doing. Then, I will ask questions about it. Ready? I will go first. I am going to pretend that I am very thirsty. I will drink some water. *With cup, pretend to drink.* What did I do? Yes, I drank water. Why did I drink water? Yes, because I was thirsty. I drank the water because I was thirsty. Please repeat that Ms. __________________ drank the water because she was thirsty. *Continue the activity, giving each child an action and a reason for action.* What did __________________ do? Why did __________________ do that? *Assist group in forming and stating complete sentences. Actions may include:*

   Pretend you are cold, and put on your coat.
   Pretend you are sleepy, put down your head, and take a nap.
   Pretend you are hungry, and eat an apple.
   Pretend you fell off your bike and hurt your arm.

2. I will give each of you a special job to do. Then, I will ask questions about it. Ready? *Whisper to each child a task to complete. Tasks may include:*

   Put all the toys on the shelf or in the box.
   Pick up all the paper on the floor.
   Push all the chairs under the table.
   Wash hands with soap.

   After all children have completed tasks, ask them: What did you do? Why did you do it? I washed my hands because they were dirty. Let's talk about our favorite things to do. I'll go first. I love to cook because I love to eat. __________________, what is your favorite thing to do? *After response:* Why is that your favorite thing to do? *Assist children in forming complete sentences if necessary. Encourage use of complete sentences.*

3. Let's talk about our favorite TV shows. *Tell children your favorite show.* My favorite show is the "__________________." *Give reason why.* I like the "__________________" because it is __________________. *Ask each child:* What is your favorite show? *After response, ask:* Why?

   Read children nursery rhymes. After each rhyme, ask: What happened? Why? *Assist where necessary.*

Materials: Illustrated nursery rhyme books

4. Let's talk about our favorite places to go. *Tell the children your favorite place.* I like to go to the zoo. *Give reason why.* I like to watch the animals play. *Ask each child:* What is your favorite place to go? *After response, ask:* Why?

5. *Read children nursery rhymes. After each rhyme ask:* What happened? Why? *Provide assistance as needed.*

6. I am going to tell you some stories, then I will ask you questions about the stories. Listen carefully. *Make up simple stories to tell, then ask "Why" question about story. Emphasize the use of complete sentences with "because" and the past tense. For example:*

   Mike ran across the yard. He tripped over a brick and fell on the ground. He cried because he hurt his knee. Why did Mike cry? *(Because he hurt his knee.)* That is right. Mike cried because he hurt his knee. *Repeat:* Mike cried because he hurt his knee.

7. Let's talk about our favorite foods. *Tell others your favorite food and the reason for your choice.* My favorite food is ice cream. I like ice cream because I can choose from many different flavors. *Ask all children.* What is your favorite food? *After response, ask:* Why?

8. I have a finger play to share. *Teach.*

   Come kitty, come kitty,
   Here's milk for you *(cup hands to make dish and extend).*
   Kitty came running *(run fingers up arm)*
   And called, "meow, meow."

   Why did the kitty come running? The kitty came running because she wanted milk. *Ask children to repeat sentence.*

9. *Ask children "Why?" questions. Possibilities include:*

   Why do we wash our hands?
   Why do we put our toys away?
   Why do we go to sleep at night?
   Why do we eat?
   Why do we walk slowly when we have cookies on a tray?

   Ask children to repeat statements (example: We wash our hands because they are dirty.).

PROGRESS CHECK

Materials: Illustrated nursery rhyme books

Read child a short nursery rhyme. Ask questions, such as: What happened? Why? Who fell down? Where did the girl go? *If first response is not a complete sentence, assist. Child must respond to two questions in complete sentences without prompt. Observe.*

Scoring:

+	Responds to two questions in complete sentences without prompt
0	Fails to respond to two questions in complete sentences without prompt

Intermediate: Level D

Activity 4: Retelling Stories

Objective: To retell story after listening to an oral presentation

Materials: Blocks — Toy car

1. *Act out a story. As you perform the actions, tell the children what is happening.* I'm going to build a tower with these blocks. *Build tall tower.* Now, I'm going to pretend I am driving my car. *Show children toy car.* I'm driving my car down the street when suddenly an evil witch casts a spell on the car. The car starts driving on its own and runs into the tower. It knocks the tower down. *Bump into the tower with the toy car, and knock down the blocks.*

   Ask the children questions about the story. What happened first in the story? What happened next? Then what happened? What happened last? *After children have answered questions:* Please tell everything that happened in the story. *Encourage use of the words "first," "next," and "last" and complete sentences.*

   Continue above procedure acting out several different stories. Possibilities include:

   Draw a picture on the board, emphasizing the order of each part drawn.
   Perform a simple task, such as sweeping the floor.

Materials:

Doll and doll clothes	Baby spoon and bowl
Pictures for a nursery tale	Cut-outs of story characters
Crayons	Tongue depressors or ice cream sticks

2. *Act out a story. As you perform the actions, tell the children what is happening. Tell the children a story about the doll. Dress the doll. Feed the doll. After the story, ask the children to tell what happened.* What happened first? What happened next? What happened last? Now, tell us the story in your own words.

   Using pictures, tell or read a nursery tale, such as "Peter Rabbit," "Three Little Pigs," or "Little Red Riding Hood." After the story, ask what happened. What happened first? What happened next? Then, what happened? What happened last? Now, tell the story in your own words. *Help in retelling, prompting if necessary. Encourage use of complete sentences.*

   Give children cut-outs of characters from the story. We will make puppets of the characters in the story. Then, we will act out the story with out puppets. Color the puppets first. *Give the children crayons. Distribute tongue depressors or ice cream sticks.* We will paste our characters to these sticks to make hand puppets. Watch me. *Demonstrate. When completed:* Now, we can act out the story using our puppets. *Retell story, encouraging children to use puppets.*

Action Pictures

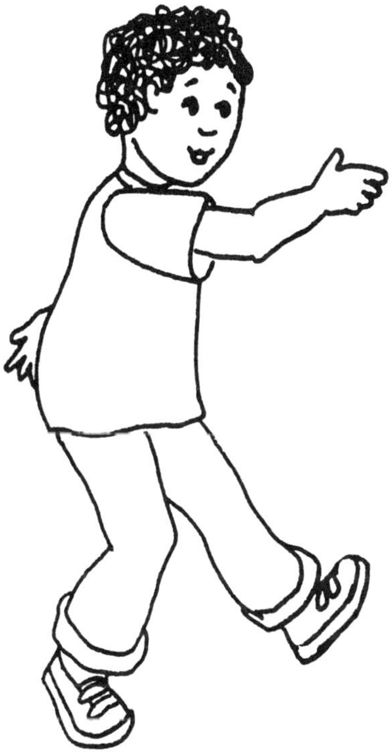

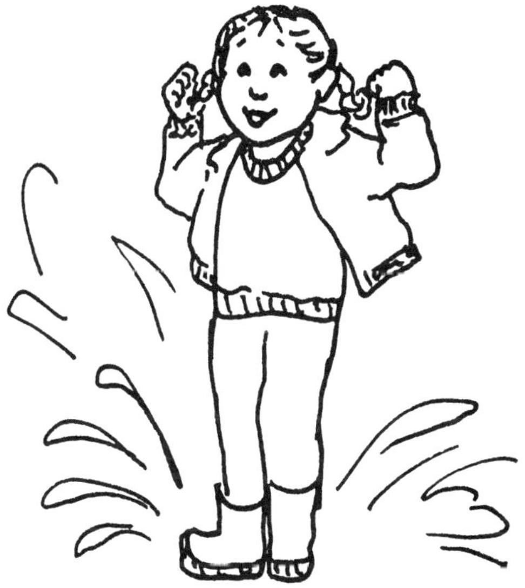

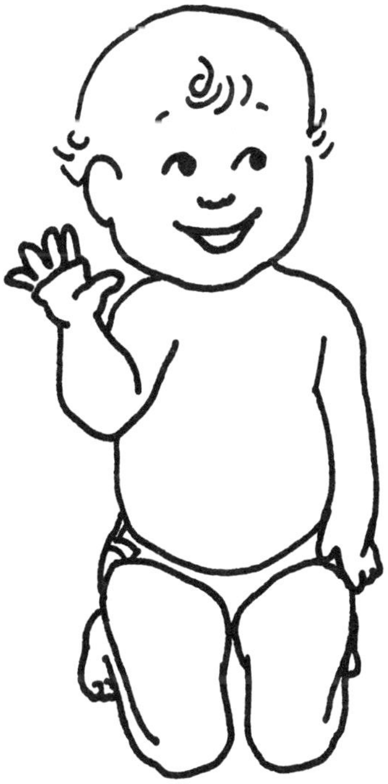

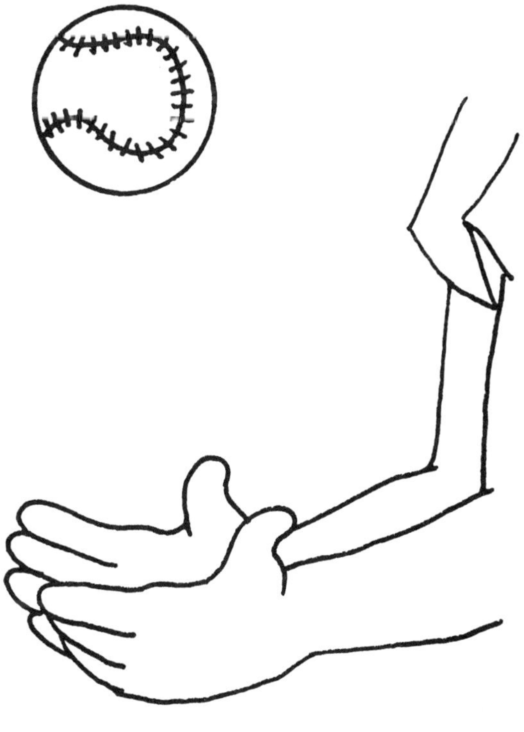

Materials: Pictures that show action

3. *Show children action picture. Tell story about picture. Then, ask children to tell what happened.* What happened first? What happened next? Then what happened? What happened last? Now, tell the story in your own words. *Prompt when necessary.*

   Show children picture of boy eating soup. Tell story:

   > Timothy was playing outside in the snow on a very cold day. He was building a snowman. He got too cold to play any longer so he went inside. His mother had a hot bowl of soup ready for him. The soup was so good, he ate it all.

   Children answer questions, then retell story.

Materials: Flannel board and cut-outs (snowman, sun, melted snowman)

4. *Using flannel board and shapes, tell children story:*

   > It was a cold winter day. Some children built a snowman *(place snowman on flannel board).* Then, the sun came out *(place sun on the board).* The snowman began to melt *(place melted snowman on board).*

   Then, ask the children to tell what happened. What happened first? What happened next? Then, what happened? What happened last? Now tell the story in your own words. *Prompt when necessary.*

Story Characters

Snow Figures and Sun

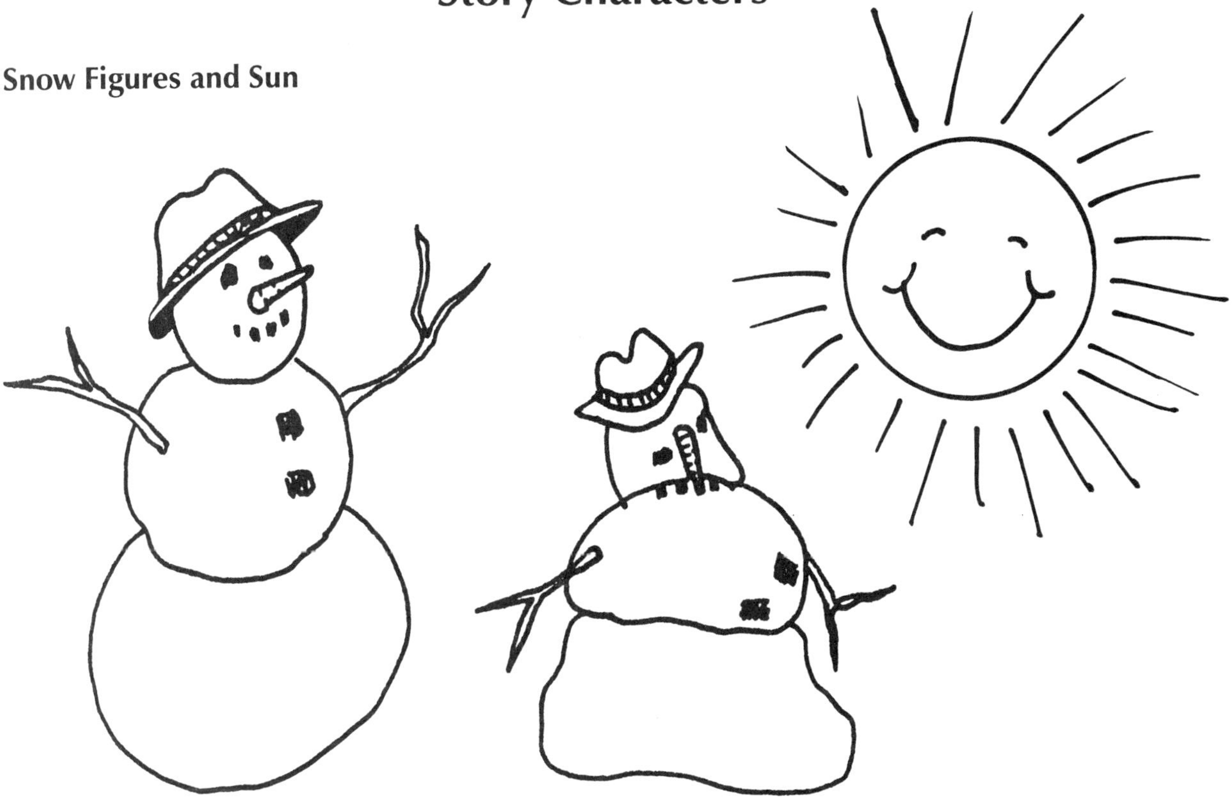

The Three Bears

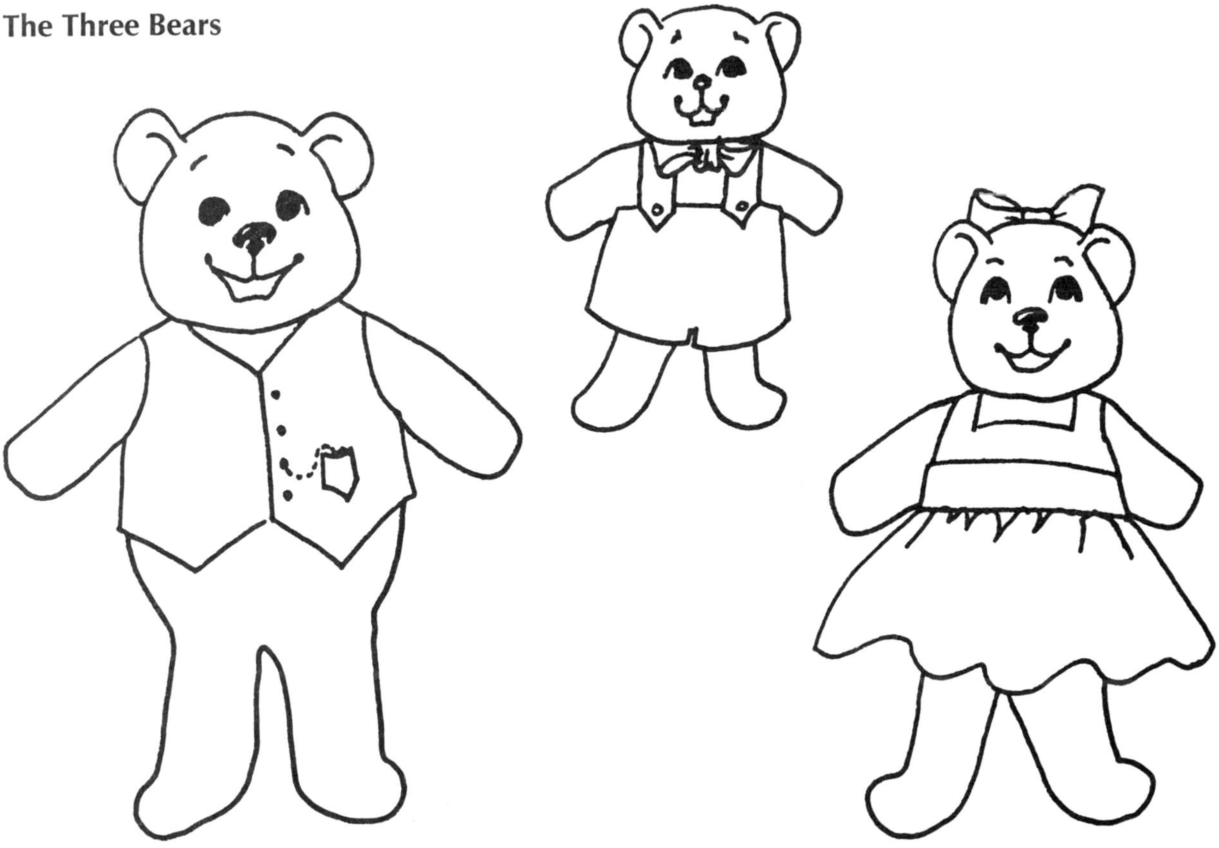

Goldilocks and the Three Bears

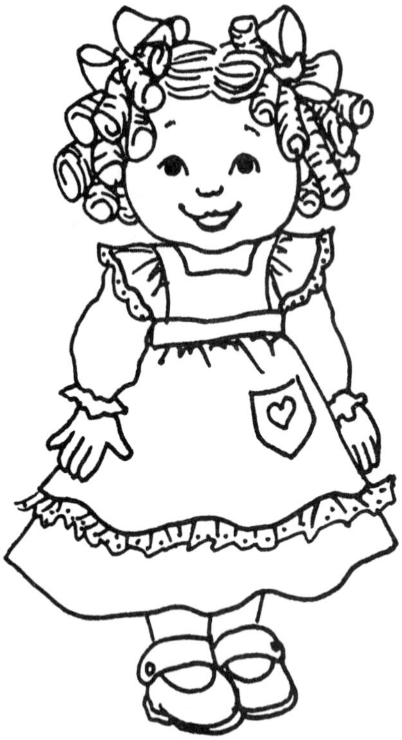

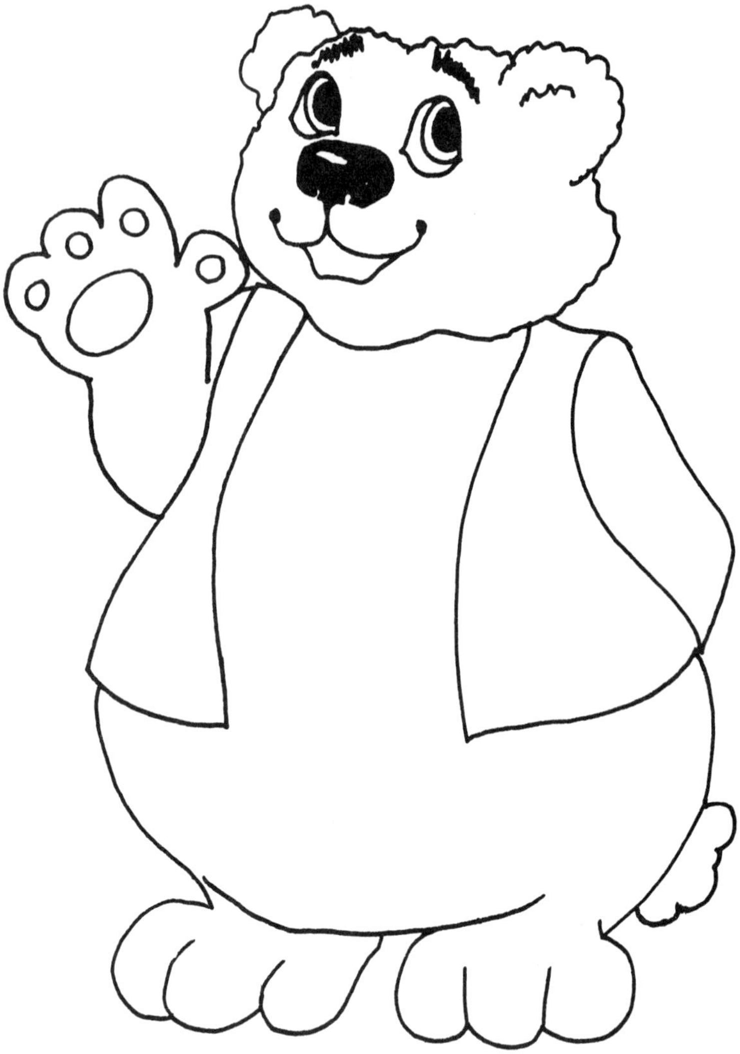

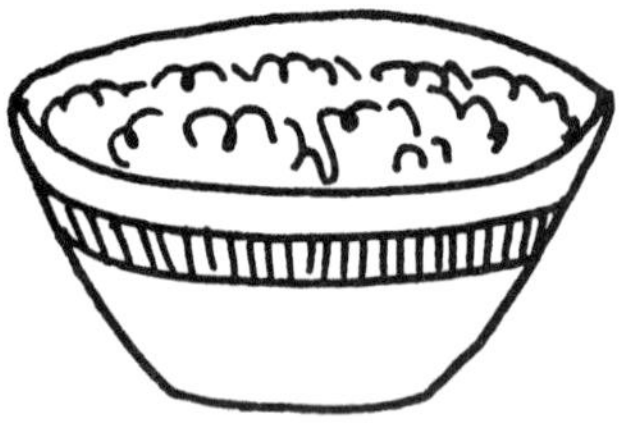

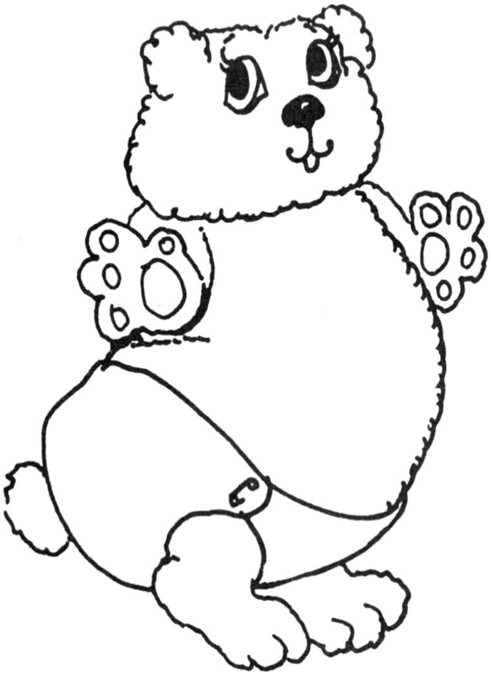

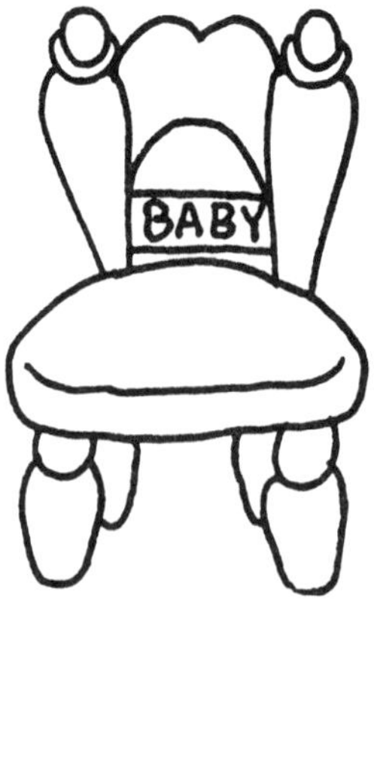

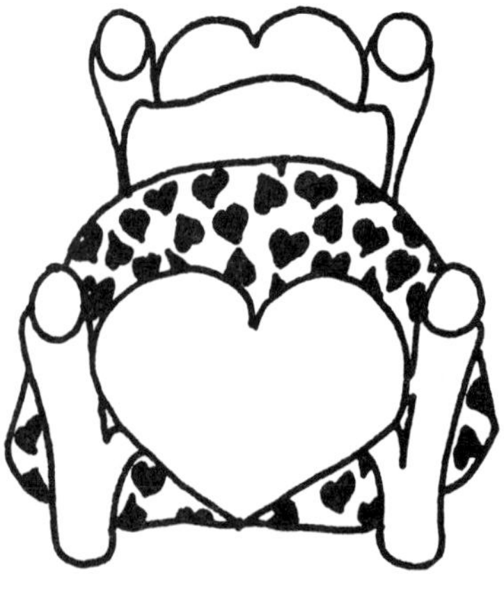

Goldilocks and the Three Bears

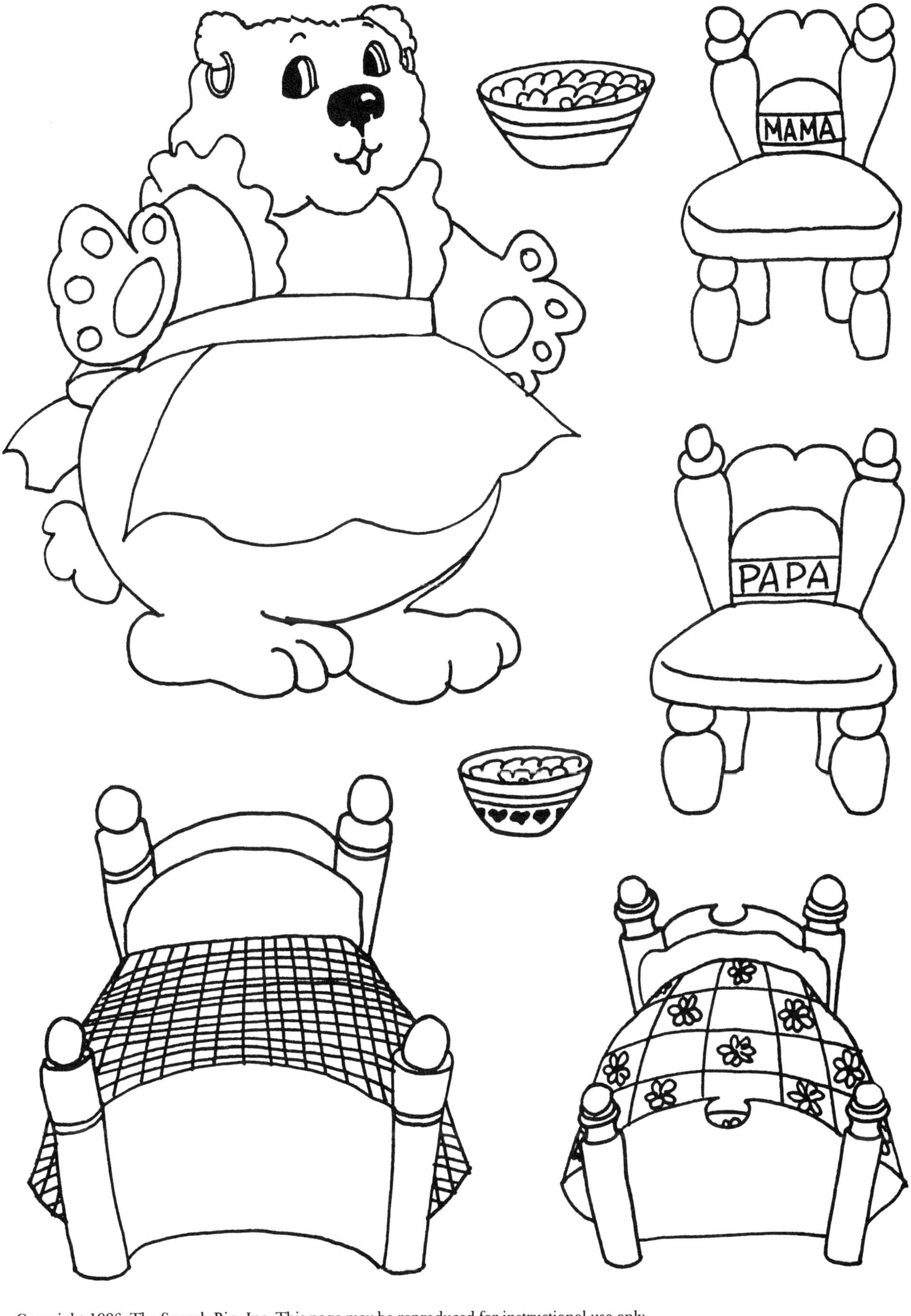

The Three Billy Goats Gruff

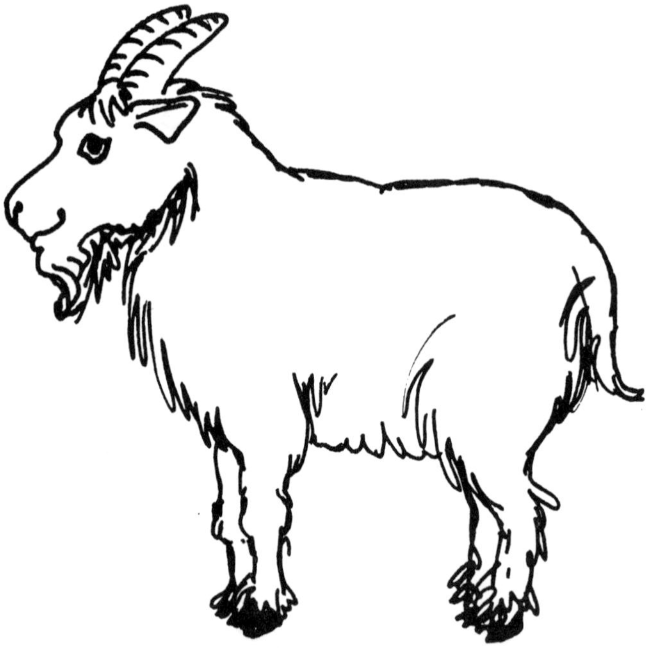

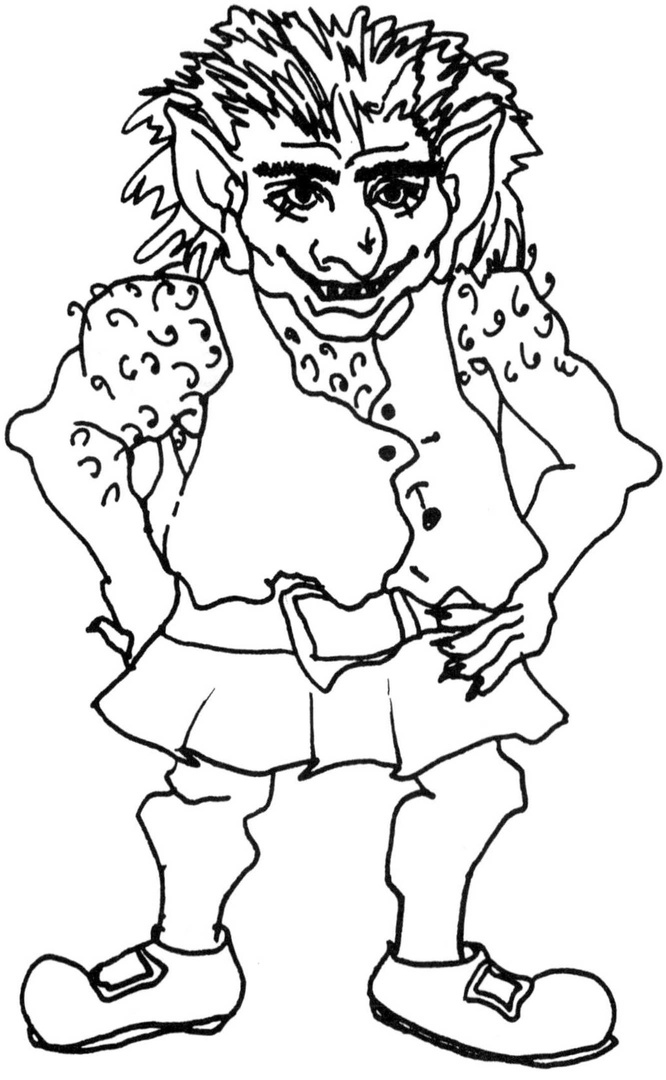

The Three Billy Goats Gruff

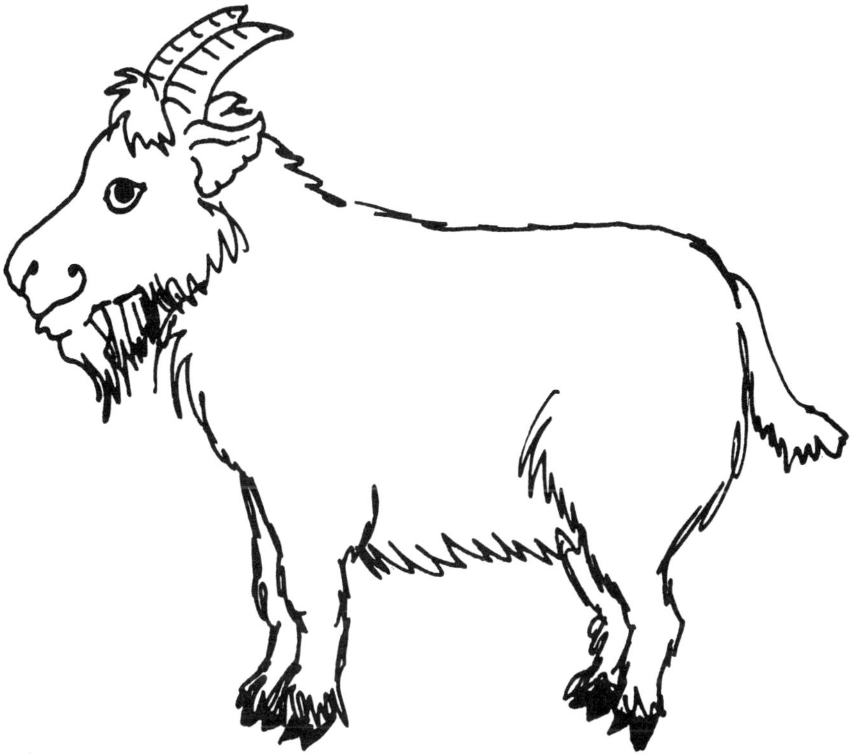

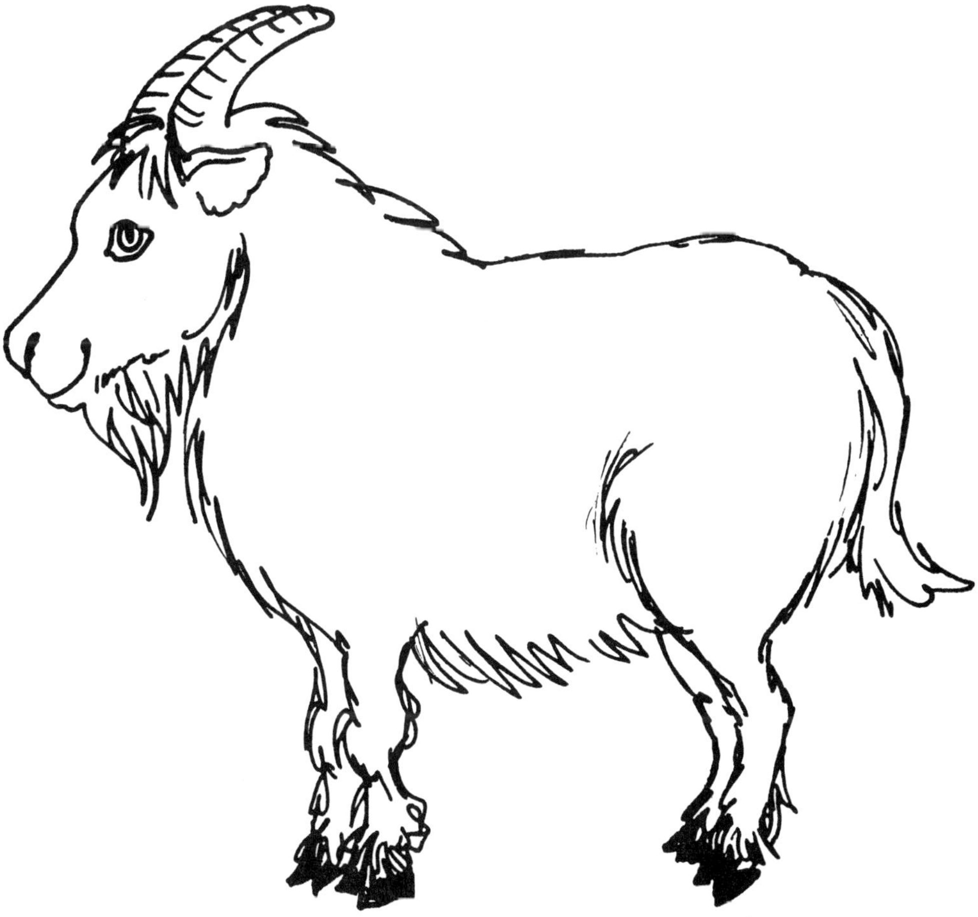

GOLDILOCKS AND THE THREE BEARS

Materials: Story of "The Three Bears"
Puppets for the story or flannel board and felt figures

5. *Using flannel board and figures, puppets or pictures, tell children story. Then ask the children to tell what happened.* What happened first? What happened next? Then what happened? What happened last? *Guide children in retelling of story. Recall story facts, using complete sentences. Ask each child to supply story facts. Possibilities include:*

Once there were three bears who lived in ________________. Because the porridge was hot they decided to ________________. While they were gone, a little girl named ________________ came to their house. The baby bear's bowl of porridge was just right, so she ________________. The baby bear's chair was just right, and it ________________. The baby bear's bed was just right, so she ________________. While she was sleeping, ________________. She was so scared by the three bears that she ________________.

THE THREE BILLY GOATS GRUFF

Materials: Story of "The Three Bill Goats Gruff"
Puppets for the story or flannel board and felt figures

6. *Using flannel board and figures, puppets, or pictures, tell children story. Then ask children to tell what happened.* What happened first? What happened next? Then what happened? What happened last? *Guide children in retelling of story. Recall story facts using complete sentences. Ask each child to supply story facts. Possibilities include:*

Once upon a time there were three billy goats who wanted to go ________________. A mean old troll lived ________________. The troll said, "Now I'm coming to ________________." The first billy goat said, "________________." The second billy goat came across the bridge. The mean old troll said, "________________." The last billy goat came across the bridge and ________________.

THE THREE LITTLE PIGS

Materials: Storybook of "The Three Little Pigs"

7. *Tell children story, reading from storybook. Then, ask them to tell what happened.* What happened first? What happened next? Then what happened? What happened last? *Guide children as they retell the story, recalling facts in complete sentences.*

PROGRESS CHECK

Materials: Simple story not previously used

Tell a story, then say: Tell what happened. *If necessary, prompt with:* What happened first? *Give no other prompts.*

Scoring:

+	Retells story in complete sentences with no or only one prompt
0	Fails to retell story in complete sentences with no or only one prompt

Intermediate: Level D

Activity 5: Recalling Facts from a Story

Objective: To recall three facts from a story read aloud

1. *Tell the following story. Then say:* Tell me three facts about the story.

   Sammy had five marbles in his hand. He was going across the park to show the marbles to his good friend, Alonsa. Before Sammy could get to Alonsa, a dog ran by and bumped into him. The marbles scattered all over the ground. Sammy was upset, but Alonsa came over and said, "Don't worry, Sammy, I will help you find your marbles." And he did.

   Follow the same procedures for the remaining activities.

2. Listen to my poem. *Read:*

   Two little apples sitting on a tree.
   Two little apples staring at me.
   I shook the tree as hard as I could.
   Down came the apples,
   Ummmm! They were good.

3. Listen to my story. *Read:*

   A boy named Joshua had a dog named Peewee that he loved very much. One day Joshua forgot to close the gate, and Peewee ran away. Joshua and his father looked all over the neighborhood for Peewee. Joshua and his father couldn't find Peewee. They were so tired from looking they decided to go home. When they got home, they found a big surprise. Peewee was at home, waiting for them!

4. Listen to my poem. *Read "Three Little Kittens."*

Three little kittens lost their mittens, and they began to cry.
"Oh, Mother dear, we sadly fear, our mittens we have lost."
"What? Lost your mittens?
You naughty kittens,
Then you shall have no pie!"

The three little kittens found their mittens, and they began to cry,
"Oh, Mother dear, see here, see here, our mittens we have found."
"What, found your mittens?
You sweet little kittens,
Then you shall have some pie!"

5. Listen to my story. *Read:*

Sadie was riding in the car with her father. They were going to the store. On the way Sadie's father drove over some broken glass by mistake. When Sadie and her father came out of the store, they saw that a tire on their car was flat. Sadie's father changed the tire, and they went home.

6. Listen to my poem. *Read:*

Old Mother Hubbard went to the cupboard
To get her poor dog a bone.
But when she got there,
The cupboard was bare,
And so the poor dog had none.

Repeat above procedure with this poem:

Hickory, dickory dock.
The mouse ran up the clock.
The clock struck one, the mouse ran down.
Hickory, dickory dock.

7. Listen to my story. *Read:*

> Once there was a little turtle who decided to take a shortcut. Instead of crawling around a hill, the turtle decided to climb over it. But the hill was too steep. He was about halfway up the hill when he slid down and landed on his back
>
> "Oh my!" he said. "How will I ever turn over? Turning over is very difficult for turtles, you see."
>
> He tried and tried, but he couldn't turn himself over. Finally, he said, "If I try hard enough, and think hard enough, I know I can turn over!" So he tried hard, and he thought hard, and, with a great push, he flipped over.

8. *Read other similar poems and stories.*

PROGRESS CHECK

Materials: None

1. *Tell child a simple story similar those used previously. For example:*

   One day a little boy named Ben went to the store to buy some candy. He reached in his pocket for his money. His pocket was empty. "Oh," cried Ben, "I forgot my money." He ran back home and found his money. It was on the table where he had left it.

   Then, say: Tell me three facts about the story.

Scoring:

+	Tells three facts with no prompts
0	Fails to tell three facts

Materials: Story of "Little Red Riding Hood"

2. *Read "Little Red Riding Hood" to child. Then, say:* Tell me three facts about the story.

Scoring:

+	Tells three facts with no prompts
0	Fails to tell three facts

Readiness: Level E

Activity 1: Categories

Objective: To name the category when shown objects

Materials: Four small tools (hammer, pliers, wrench, screwdriver)
Four items that are *not* tools
Large bag, box, or tool box

1. We are going to talk about tools. Tools are instruments we use to help with a job. Look at some of the tools I have here. *Hold up hammer.* What is this? Yes, it is a hammer. A hammer is a tool. We use a hammer to hit nails. *Continue, holding up and identifying each tool. Discuss use of each. Ask:* What tools do you have at your house?

   Put items and box on table. Let's play "Bag It." Select an item from this pile. If the item is a tool, put it in the tool box (or bag). If item is not a tool, put the item here on the table. *Indicate place.* Ready? *Call on each child to select items from the pile and sort accordingly.*

   Let's look at the things we put in the tool box. *Remove items from box and ask children to identify each one.* Let's see how many kinds of tools we can name. I will keep count. *As children name items, count them aloud.*

Materials: Four items of clothing
Four small tools (hammer, pliers, wrench, screwdriver)
Large bag
Large bag, box, or tool box

2. We have talked about tools. Tools are instruments we use to help do a job. Today, we are going to talk about clothes. Clothes are things we wear. Look at my clothes. *Name items being worn, and point to each one.* I am wearing a dress and a pair of shoes. Because the weather was cool this morning, I wore my sweater. Now, let's look at the clothes you are wearing. *Ask each child to name items of clothing worn.*

   Put items, bag, and box on table. Let's play "Bag It." Select an item from this pile. If the item is a tool, put it in the tool box. If the item is clothing, put it in the clothes bag. Ready? *Allow each child the opportunity to select item from pile, and sort accordingly.*

   Let's look at the things we put in the tool box. *Remove items from the box, and ask children to identify each one. Continue with the clothes bag.* Let's see how many kinds of clothes we can name.

Materials: Eight pictures of people (four children and four adults)

3. *Show pictures to the children; personalize statements to your pictures.* Look at these pictures of people. *Hold up picture.* What do you see? Yes, this is a picture of an old man. The old man has white hair and glasses. *Show the next picture to children.* Look at this picture. What do you see? Yes, this is a picture of a little girl. She has braids, and she is missing a tooth. *Continue, introducing each picture.* These pictures are pictures of people. Who are some of your favorite people? *Allow each child the opportunity to respond.*

   Lay pictures face up on table. All these pictures are pictures of people. Some pictures are of older people or adults. Some are of younger people or children.

   > ____________________, find a picture of a child. We will put the pictures of the children here. *Indicate the appropriate place for the pictures.* ____________________, can you find a picture of an older person or an adult? We will put the pictures of the adults over there. *Indicate place.*
   >
   > Select a picture. Tell if the picture is of a child or an adult, then put the picture in the appropriate pile. *Ask each child to participate.*

Materials: Four pictures each of people, kinds of transportation, tools, and clothing

4. *Show children pictures of people.* These are pictures of people. We are all people. *Present each picture, and discuss its content.* Who are some other people we know?

   Show children pictures of kinds of transportation. These are pictures of kinds of transportation – things we can ride in.

   Present each picture and discuss its content. What kinds of transportation have you ridden?

   > I am going to mix up the pictures of people and transportation, and put them here so you can see them. *Display pictures.* Select a picture, and tell what it is. Say: "This is a picture of people, or this is a picture of a kind of transportation."

   Point to the pictures of the people. Indicate what the picture is.

   I am going to mix up the pictures of people and transportation with the pictures of clothing and tools. *Put pictures on table.*

   You choose a picture, tell if the picture is a picture of transportation, clothing, tools or people, and then put the picture on the bottom of the pile.

People: Children

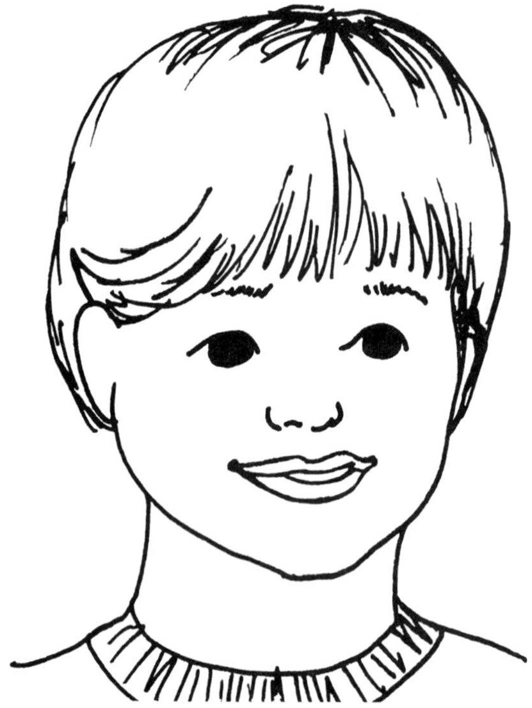

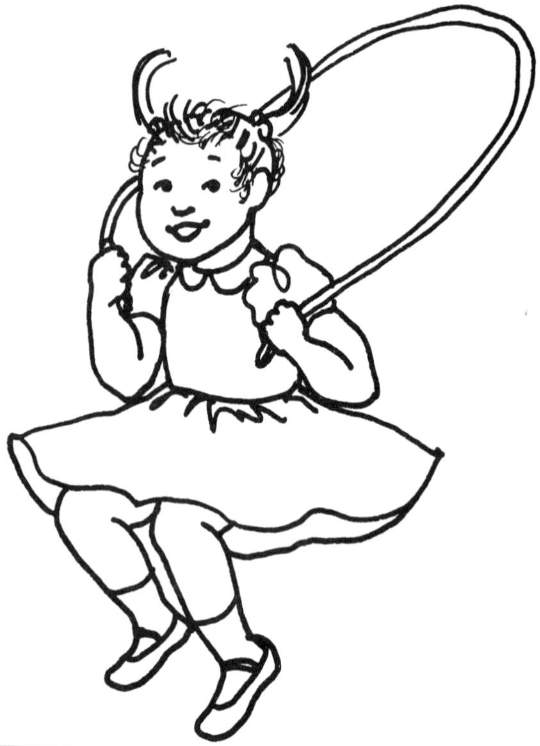

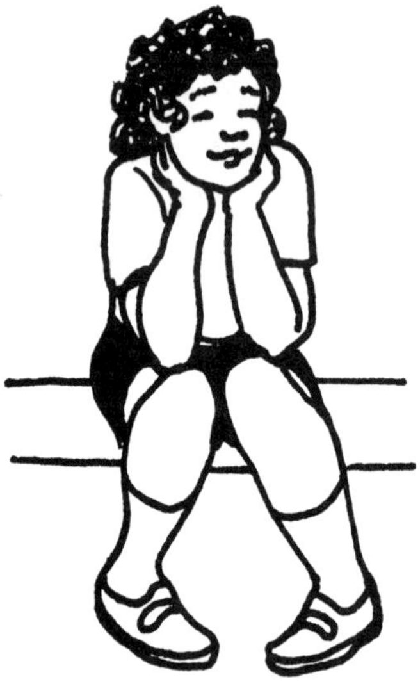

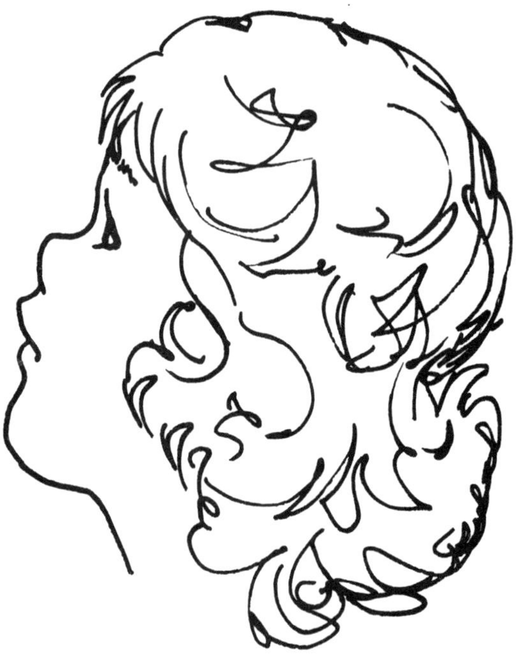

People: Adults

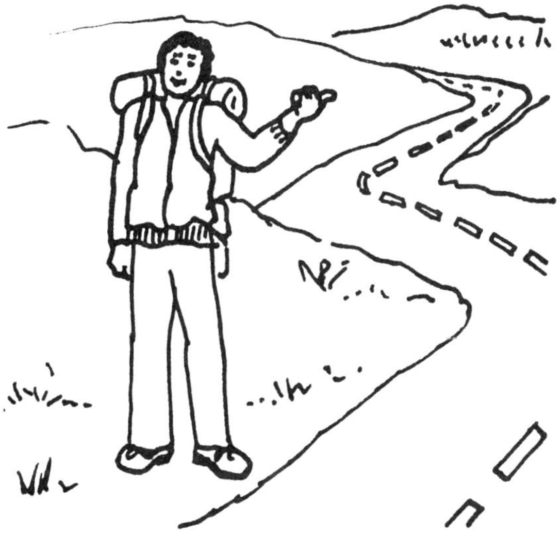

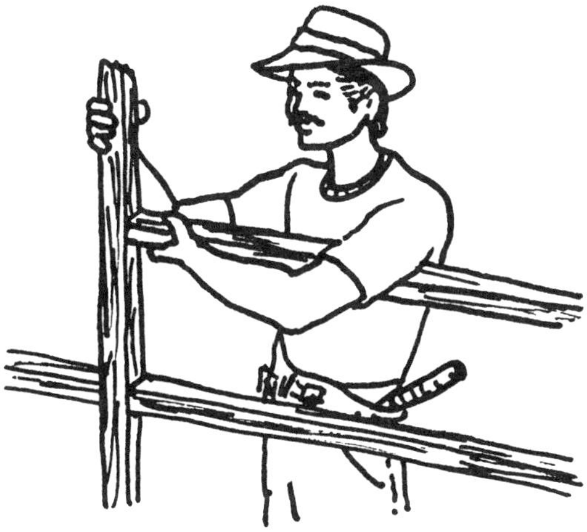

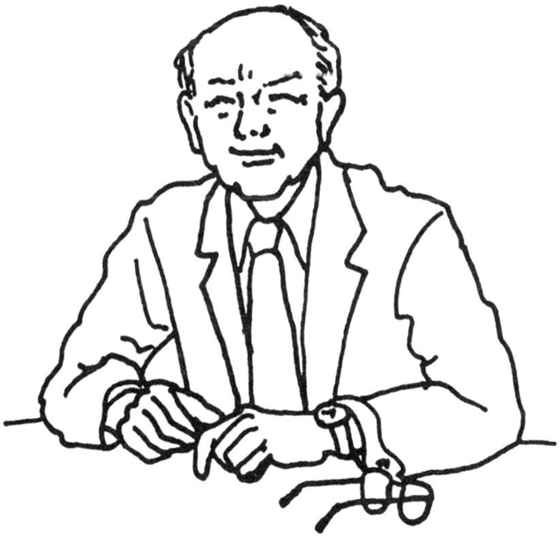

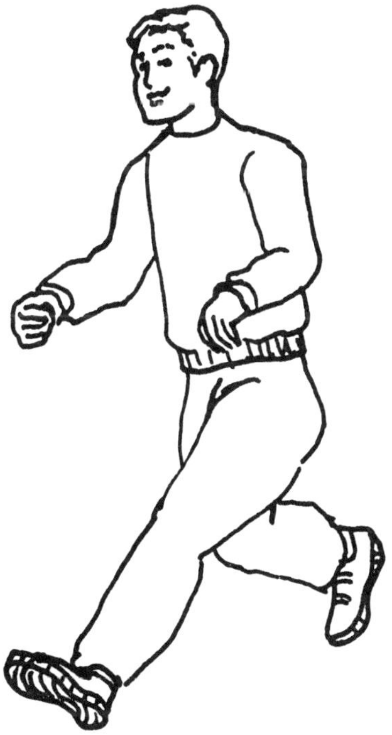

Transportation

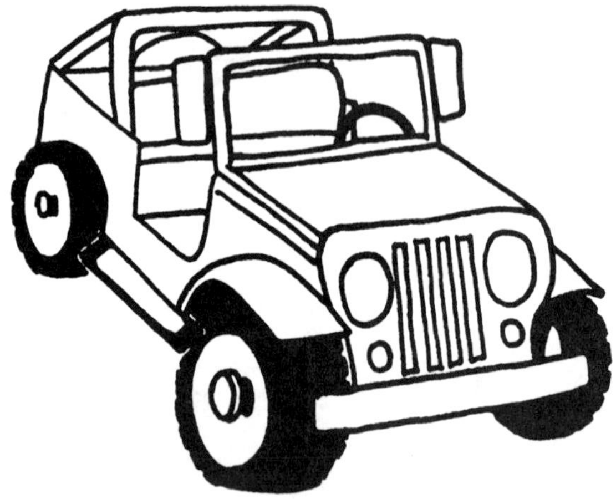

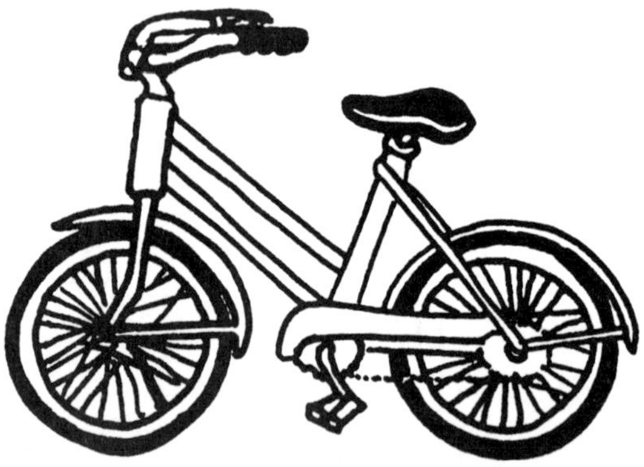

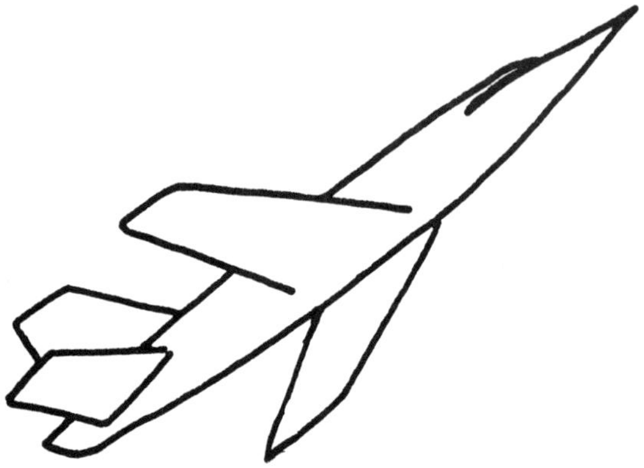

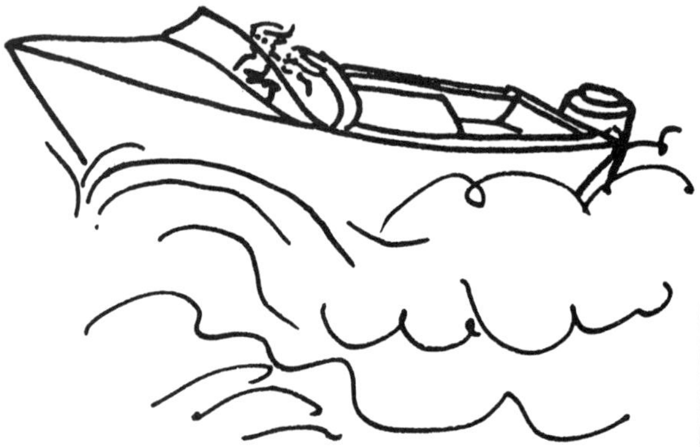

Tools

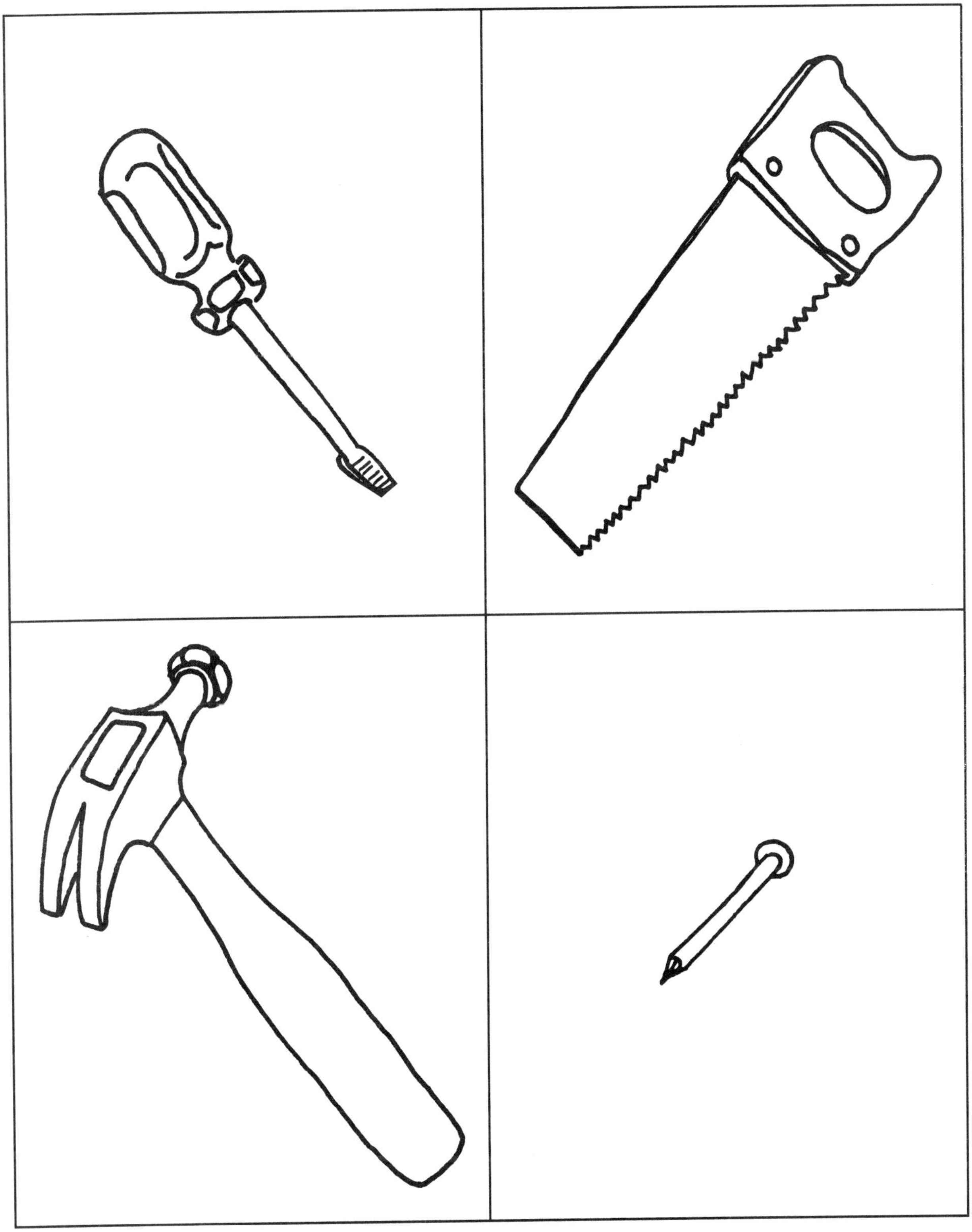

Clothing

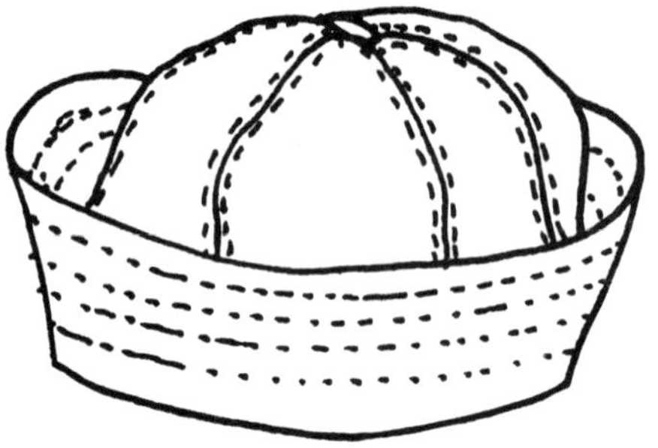
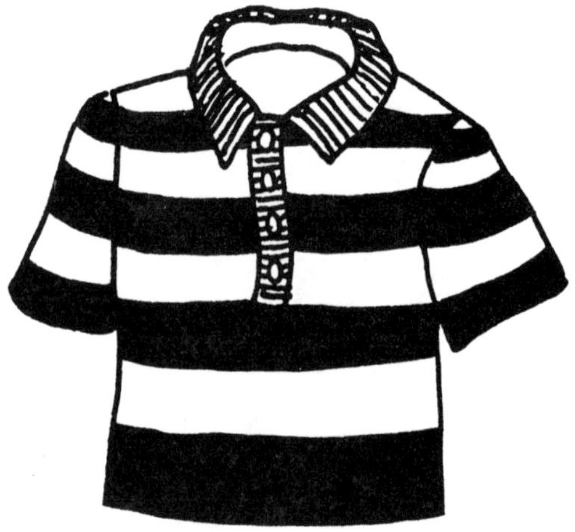
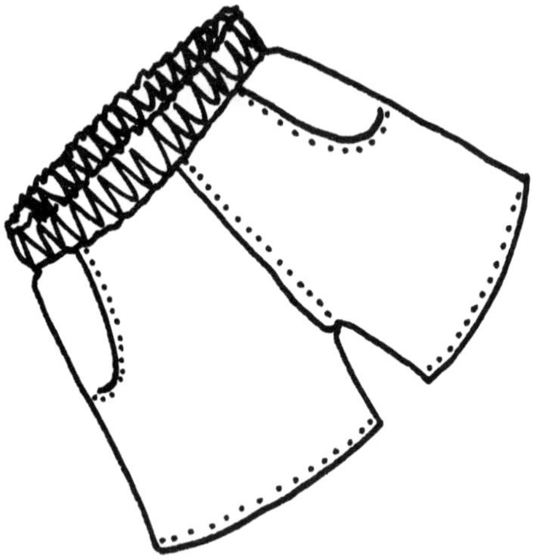
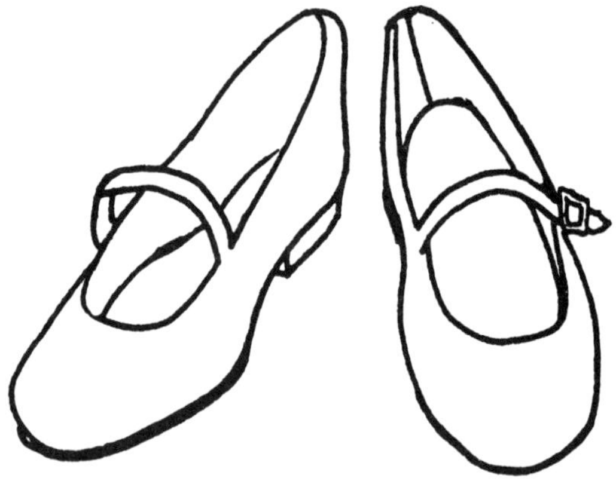
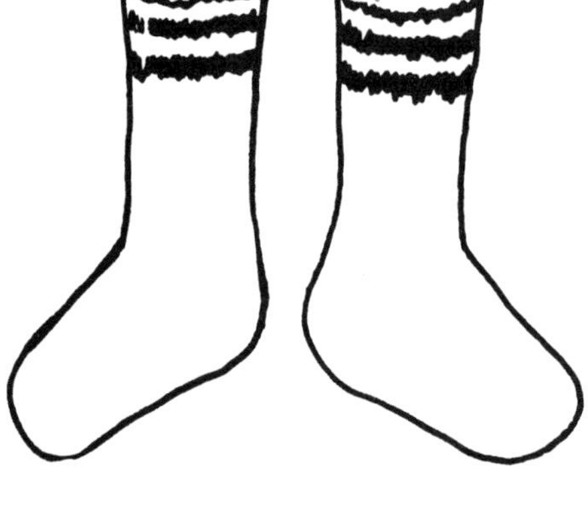
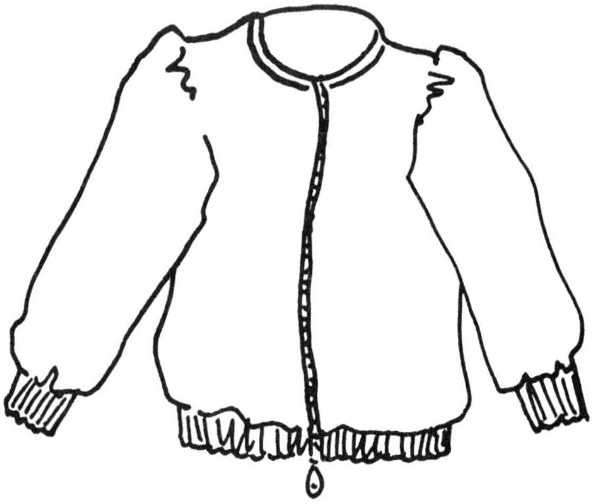

Materials: Five pictures each of animals and plants

5. *Show children pictures of animals.* These are pictures of animals. *Present each picture, and discuss its content.* What are your favorite animals?

   Show children pictures of plants. These are pictures of plants. *Present each picture, and discuss its content.* What kinds of plants do you have at home? *If possible, go to window or outside doorway.* What plants do you see outside?

   I am going to mix the pictures of animals and plants. I will put them on the table so you can see them. *Display the pictures.* Choose a picture, and tell what it is. Say: "This is an animal," or "This is a plant." Put the pictures of the animals here. *Indicate place.* Put the pictures of the plants here. *Indicate place. Allow each child to respond.*

Materials: Five pictures each of furniture and body parts

6. *Show children pictures of furniture.* These are pictures of furniture. We have furniture in this room and in our homes. *Present each picture, and discuss its content.* What furniture do you see in this room?

   Show children pictures of body parts. These are pictures of parts of our bodies. *Present each picture, and discuss its content.* What other body parts do we have?

   I am going to mix up the pictures of furniture and parts of our bodies and put them on the table so you can see them. *Put pictures on table.* Choose a picture, and tell what it is. Say, "This is a body part, or this is furniture." Put the pictures of the body parts here. *Indicate place.* Put the pictures of the furniture here. *Indicate place. Ask each child to participate. Repeat activity, but this time mix pictures with those of animals and plants.*

Materials: Five pictures each of land features and water areas
Selected pictures of animals, plants, furniture, body parts used previously

7. *Show children pictures of land features.* These are pictures of places on the land. *Present each picture, and discuss its content.* What places have you visited?

   Show children pictures of water areas. These are pictures of water areas. *Present each picture, and discuss its content.* What kinds of water areas have you visited?

   I am going to mix up the pictures of land and water and put them on the table so you can see them. *Put pictures on table.* Choose a picture, and tell what it is. Say, " This is a picture of land, or this is a picture of water." We will put the pictures of land here and the pictures of water here. *Indicate places.*

   Repeat this activity by adding pictures used previously (animals, plants, furniture, body parts).

Animals

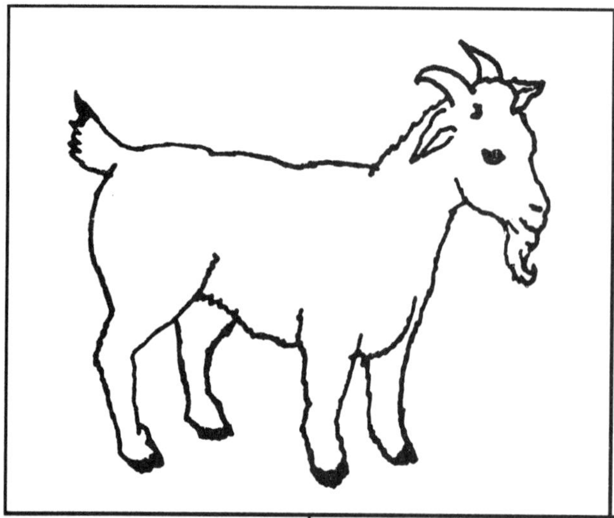

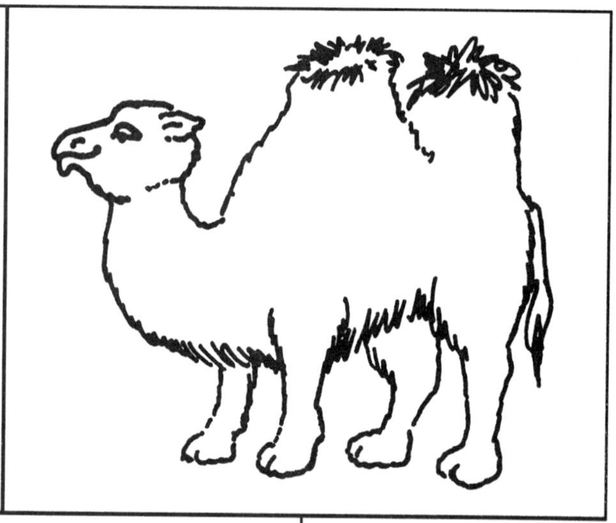

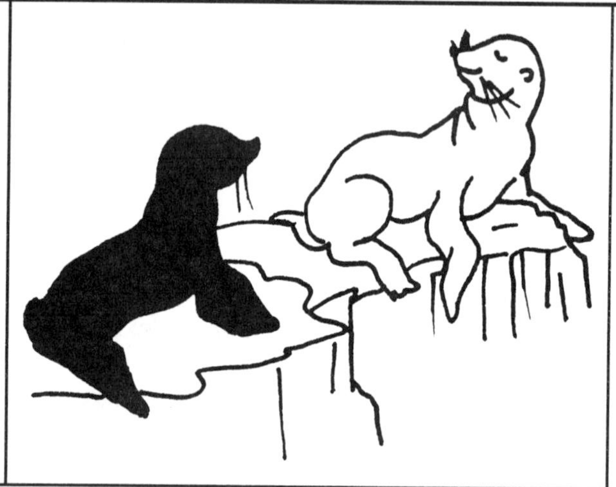

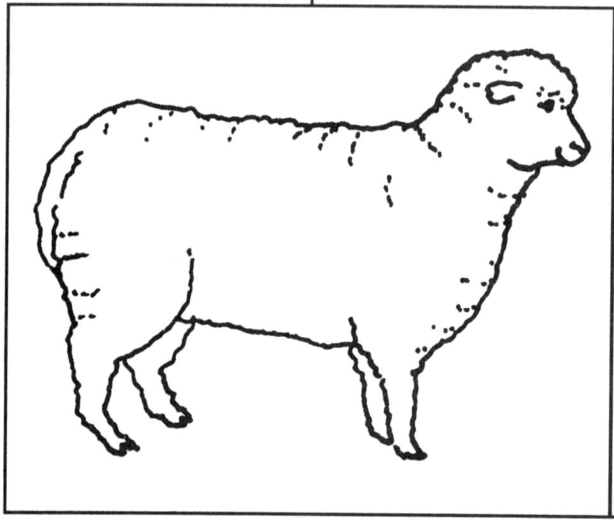

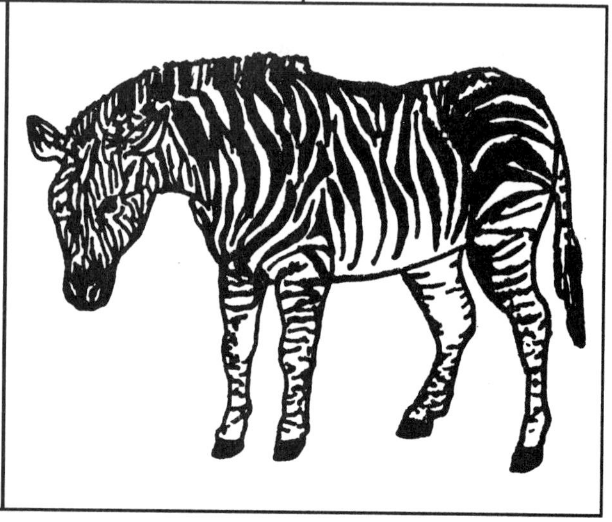

Plants

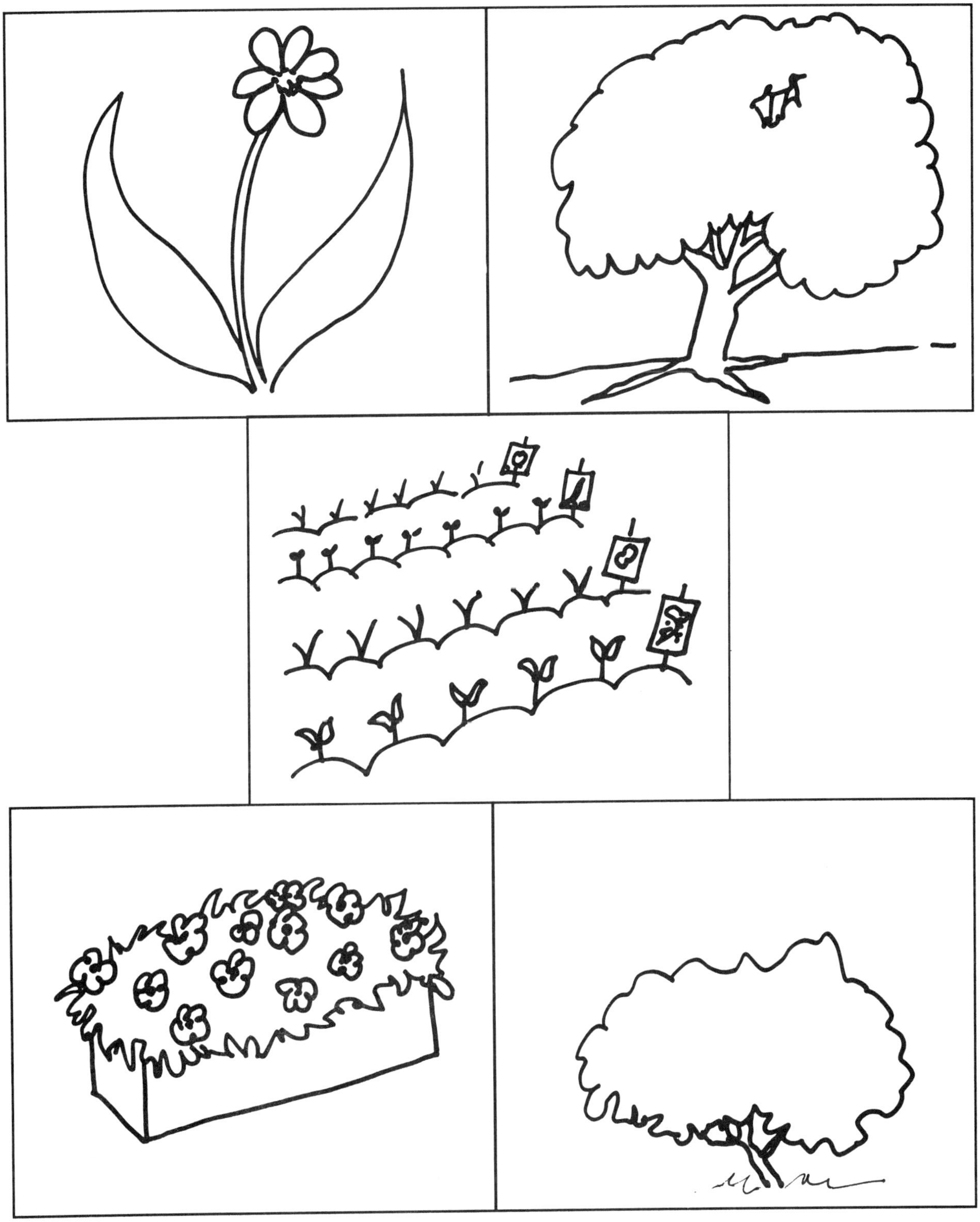

Furniture

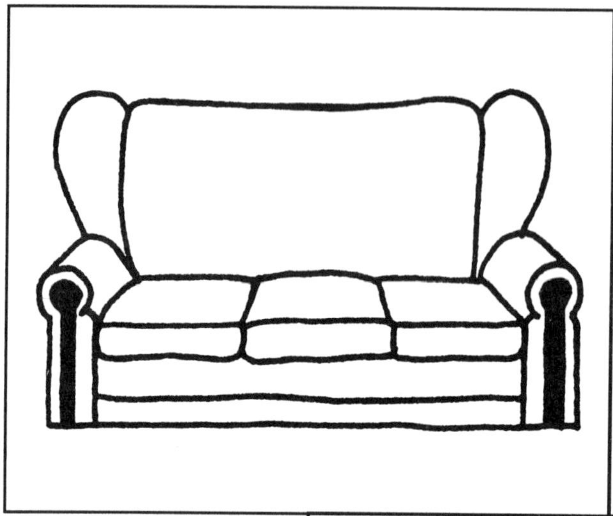

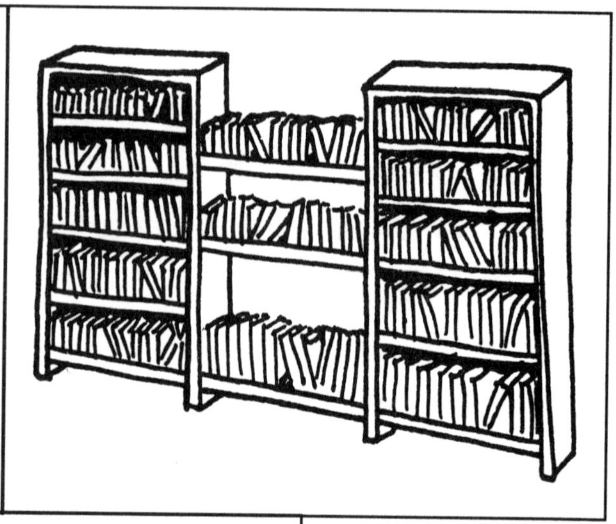

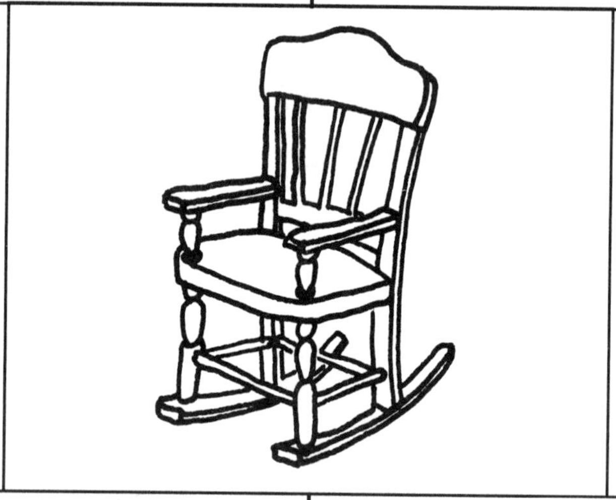

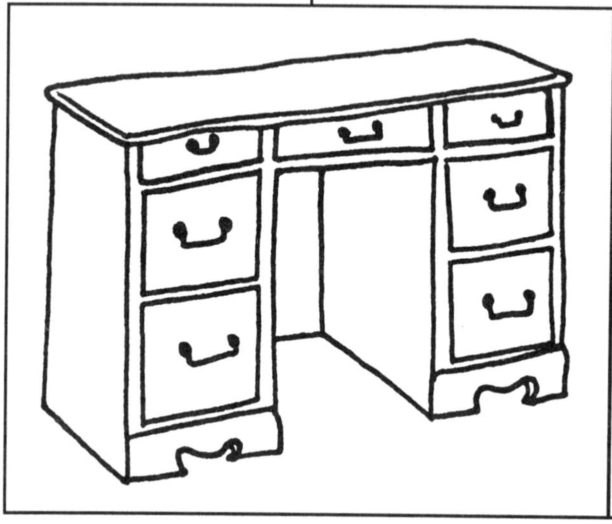

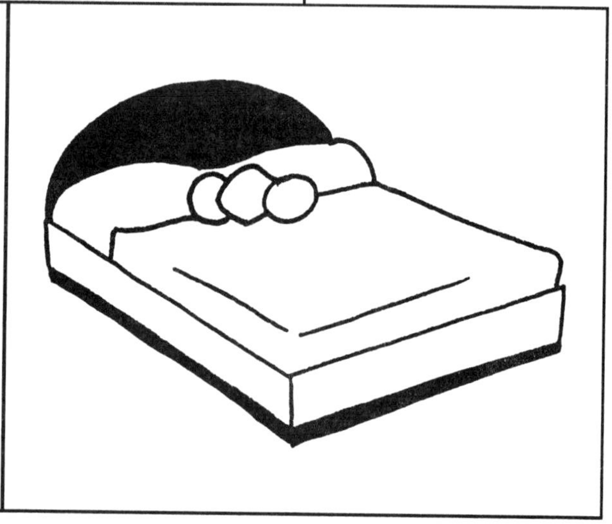

Parts of the Body

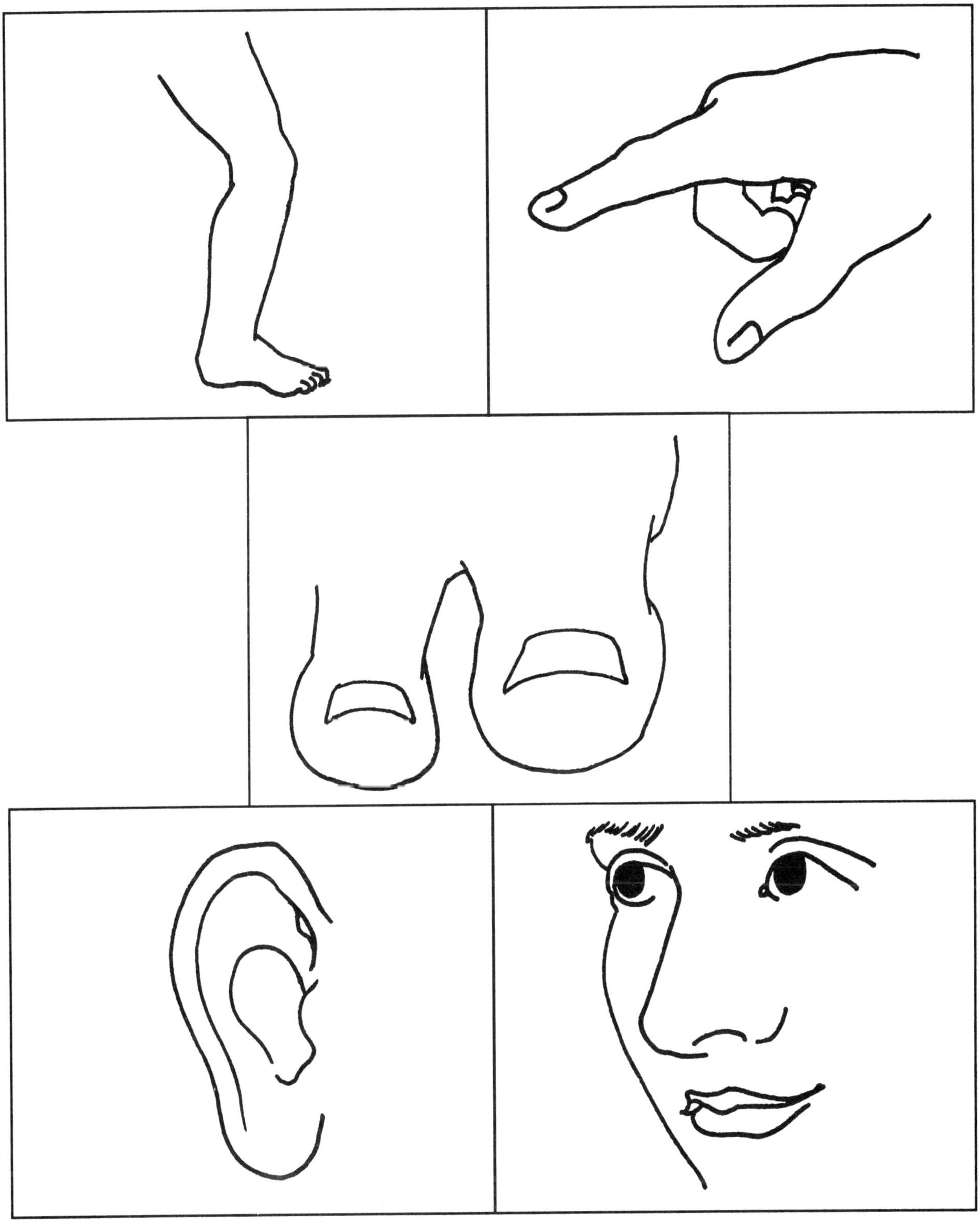

Bodies of Water

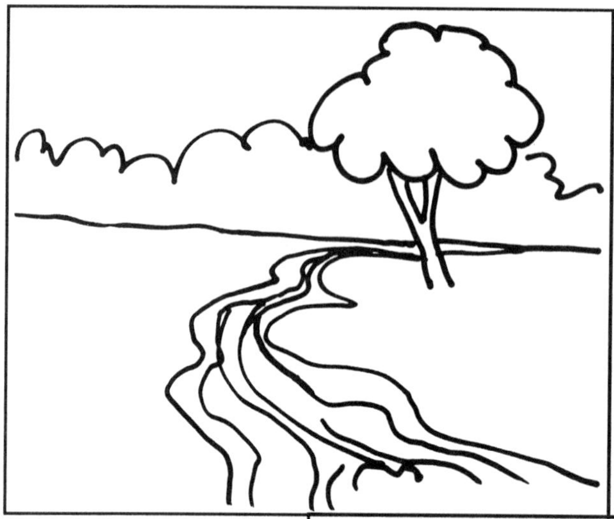

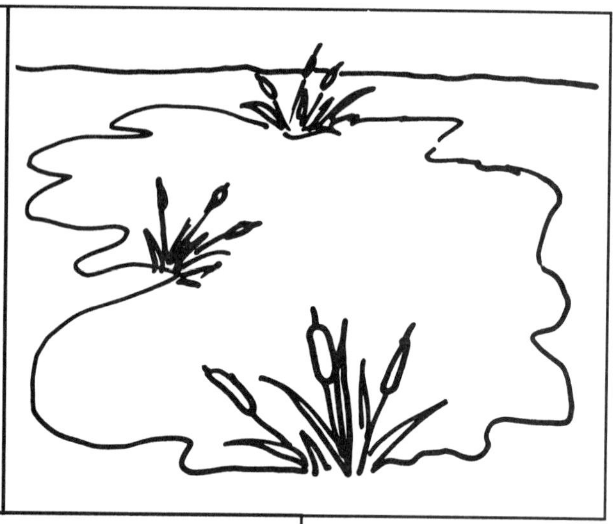

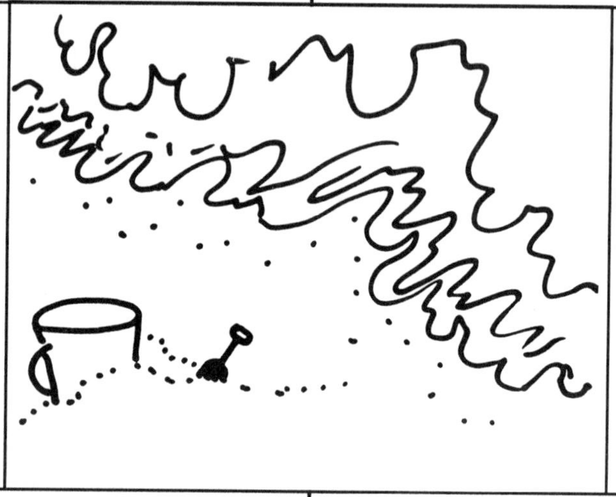

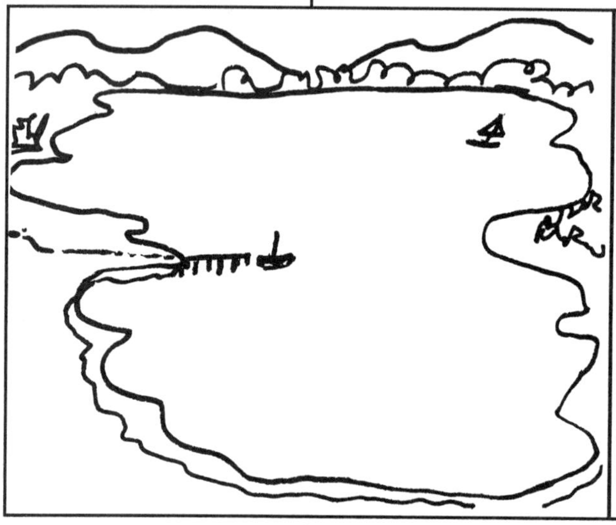

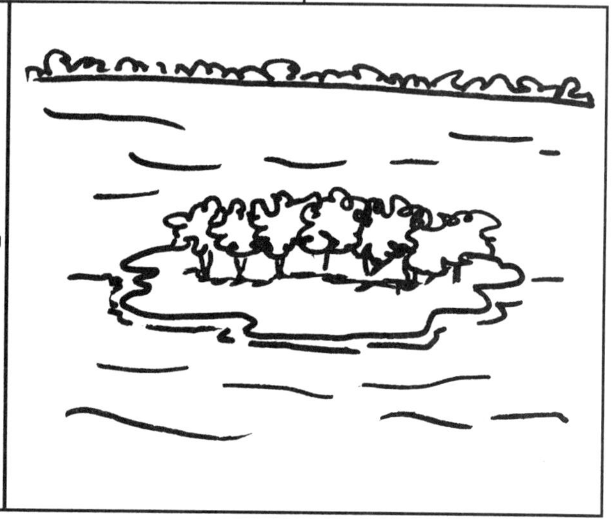

Land Features

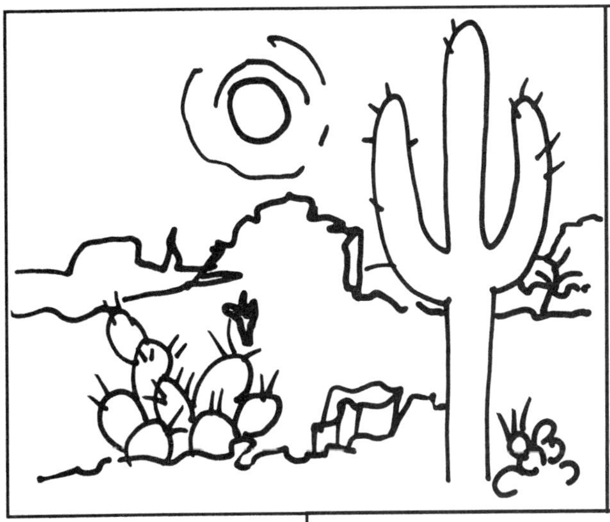
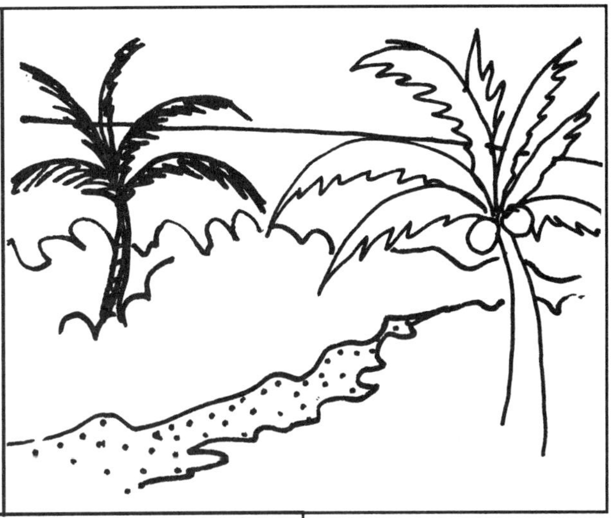
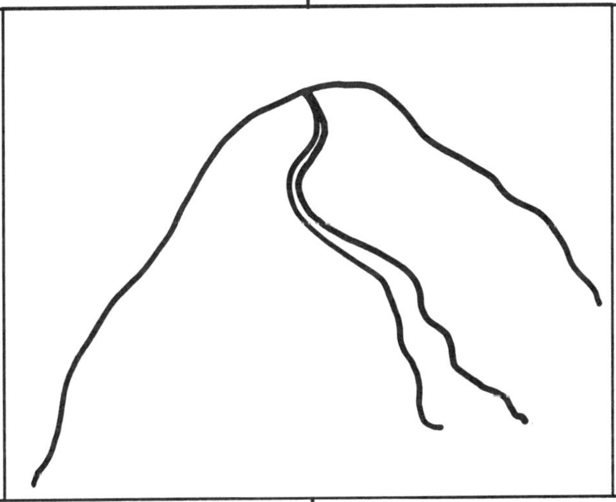
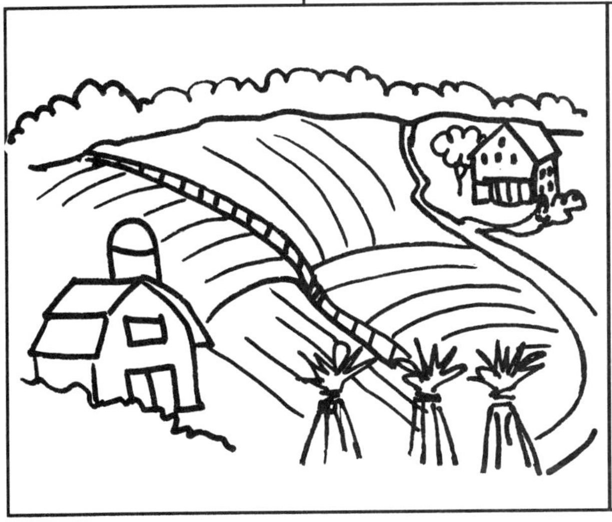
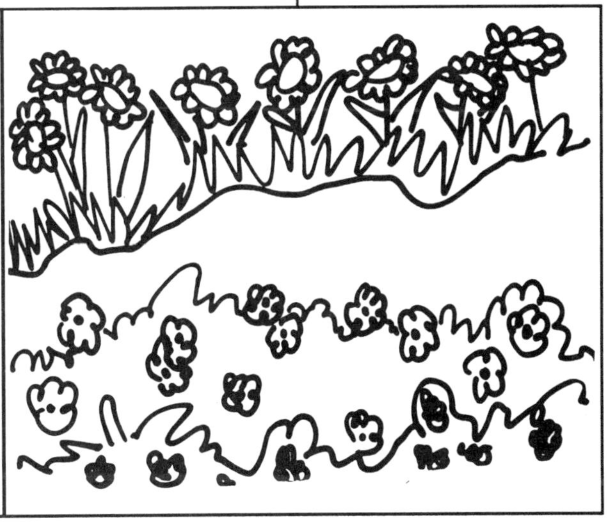

Materials: Five pictures each of –

Bodies of water	Land features
Animals	Plants
Furniture	Parts of the body

8. *Place pictures on table.* Let's play "Name and Sort." *Hold up picture of people.* This picture shows people. I will put the picture here. *Indicate place.*

   Continue activity, showing one picture from each category (animals, plants, furniture, parts of the body, land features, and bodies of water), and indicating appropriate positions on table.

   Place remaining pictures in a stack in front of the children. Choose a picture from the top of the pile. Show the picture, and tell if it shows animals, plants, furniture, parts of the body, land features, or bodies of water, then put the picture in the correct place. Ready?

   Ask each child to select a picture, show it to the others, identify category, and sort.

PROGRESS CHECK

Materials: Four pictures each of people, kinds of transportation, animals, plants, water areas, land features, tools, clothing

1. *Place pictures on table (three from each category): people, kinds of transportation, animals, plants, land features, tools, clothing, and water areas.*

2. *Ask child to choose picture, identify the category, and select the other pictures belonging to that category. Follow this procedure for all categories.*

Scoring:

+	Identifies six categories and selects pictures in each category
0	Fails to identify six categories and select pictures in each category

Readiness: Level E

Activity 2: Opposites

Objective: To name opposites

ON and OFF

Materials: Flashlight Book

1. *Introduce concepts "on" and "off." Begin by using the light switch in the classroom.* We are going to talk about on and off. Look at the lights. *Point to ceiling lights.* The lights in this room are on. Now watch. *Turn the lights off.* Now, the lights are off. Watch again. *Turn the lights on.* Now, the lights are on. *Turn the lights off.* Now, the lights are off. "On" and "off" are opposites. Are the lights on or off? *Turn lights on and off several times.*

   Show flashlight to the children. This is a flashlight. It helps people see in the dark. If I push this button, the light will come on. *Demonstrate.* The light is on. Now, I push the button again, and the light goes off. *Demonstrate.* The light is off. We say, "The light is on *(turn on)* or off" *(turn off)*. Now, you try. Turn the light on, and say, "The light is on." Then, turn the light off, and say, "The light is off." *Ask each child to participate.*

   Look at my shoes. They are on my feet. *Take one shoe off.* Look, I have one shoe on *(point). Ask each child to point to a shoe that is on or off.* ________________, point to the shoe that is on. ________________, point to the shoe that is off. *Continue asking each individual child to identify "on" or "off."*

   Place a book on the table. The book is on the table. *Place the book on a chair or the floor.* The book is off the table. *Put the book on the table.* Where is the book? Yes, it is on the table. *Put the book on the floor.* Where is the book now? Yes, it is off the table. *Move book, and ask each child to tell if the book is "on" or "off" the table.*

OLD and NEW, DIRTY and CLEAN

Materials: Sets of objects that are "old" and "new," such as crayons, books, pencils
Sets of objects that are "dirty" and "clean," such as a cloth or piece of paper
Pictures of "old" and "new" objects
Pictures of "dirty" and "clean" objects

2. *Put "old" and "new" materials on the table. Show children an old crayon.* This is an old crayon. *Show them a new crayon.* This is a new crayon. *Continue for other sets of objects. Then, say:* "Old" and "new" are opposites. Please choose an item from this pile, and tell if it is old or new. *Allow each child a turn.* Now, I want you to select one item from this pile, tell if it is old or new, then find its opposite. *Ask each child to participate.*

Put "dirty" and "clean" objects on table. Show the children a dirty cloth. This cloth is dirty. *Show them a clean cloth.* This cloth is clean. *Continue displaying other objects. Then say:* "Dirty" and "clean" are opposites. Choose an item from this pile, and tell if it is dirty or clean. *Lay pictures of "dirty" and "clean" and "new" and "old" items on the table.* Select a picture, and tell if it is dirty or clean or old or new.

WET and DRY, HOT and COLD

Materials: Pictures to illustrate "wet" and "dry," "hot" and "cold"

3. *Introduce pictures of "wet" and "dry." Discuss these concepts.* These pictures show things that are wet or dry. Choose a picture, and tell if it is wet or dry. We'll put the wet pictures here and the dry pictures there. *Indicate appropriate places.*

   Introduce pictures of "cold" and "hot." Discuss these concepts. These pictures show things that are cold or hot. Choose a picture, and tell if it is cold or hot. We'll put the cold pictures here and the hot pictures there.

   Display "wet" and "dry" and "cold" and "hot" pictures. These pictures show things that are wet or dry and things that are hot or cold. Choose a picture, and tell if it is something wet or dry or something hot or cold, then put the picture in the appropriate pile.

ABOVE and BELOW

Materials: Flannel board
Two each of several objects, such as umbrella, apple, star, ball (page 29)
Balls (can be made of masking tape and crumpled newspaper)

4. *Review concepts "on" and "off" using flannel board.* I will put the star on the board. Now I will take the star off. *Repeat actions.* Where is the car? Now, where is the car? *Introduce concepts "above" and "below."* The star is on the board. I will put the star above the car. I will put the ball below the car. Where is the star? Yes, the star is above the car. Where is the ball? The ball is below the star. *Remove cut-outs.* I have put the apple on the board. *Place star above the apple.* Where have I put the star? *Move star below apple.* Where is the star now? *As objects are moved, ask each child to participate.*

   Place one cut-out on the board. Give each child a cut-out. ____________________, put your cut-out on the board below the star. *Continue until all children have placed their cut-outs on the flannel board.*

   After all cut-outs are on the flannel board, ask children questions, such as: Where did

   ____________________ put the cut-out? ____________________, where did you put

   your cut-out?

Opposites: Old and New, Clean and Dirty, Wet and Dry

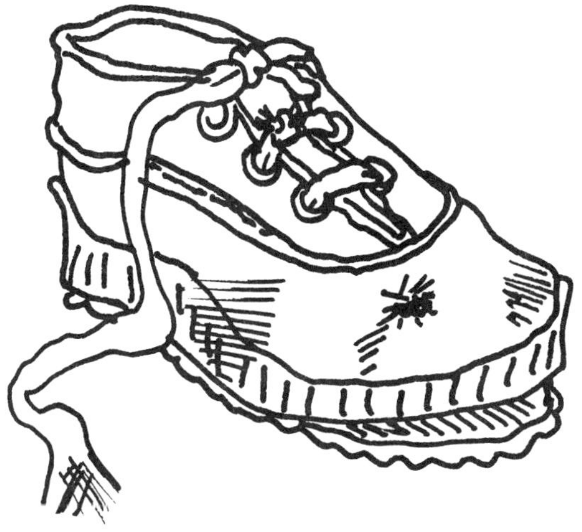

old

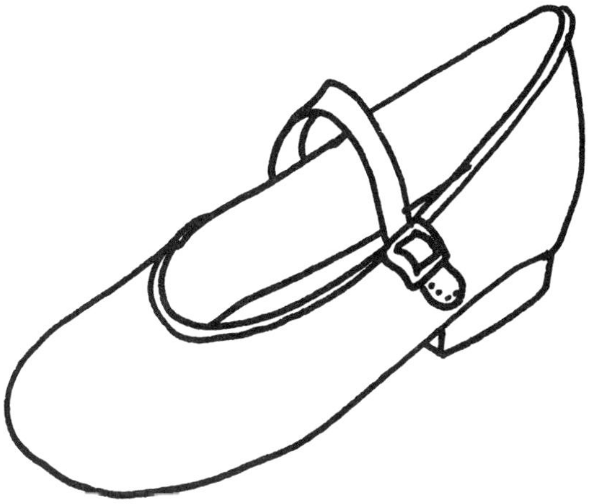

new

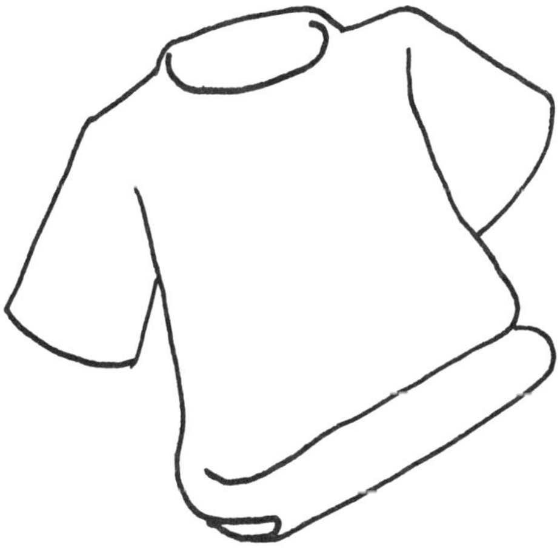

clean

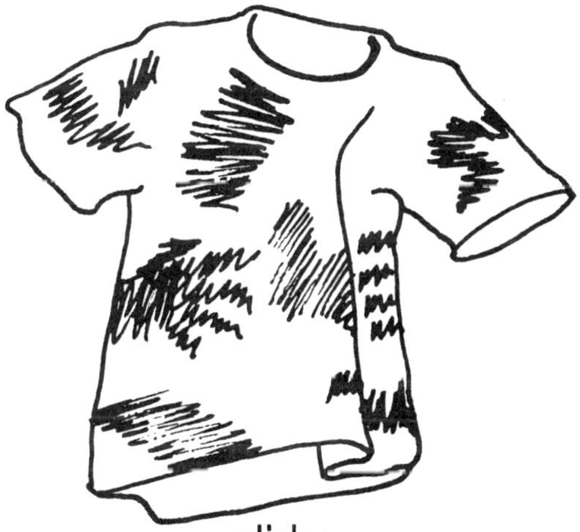

dirty

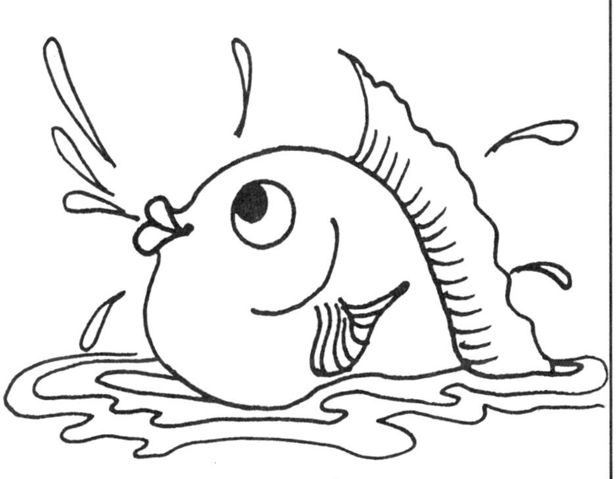

wet

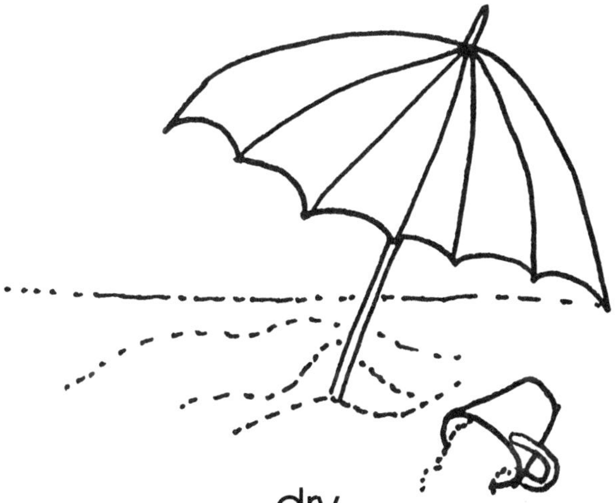

dry

Opposites: Open and Shut, Fast and Slow, Hot and Cold

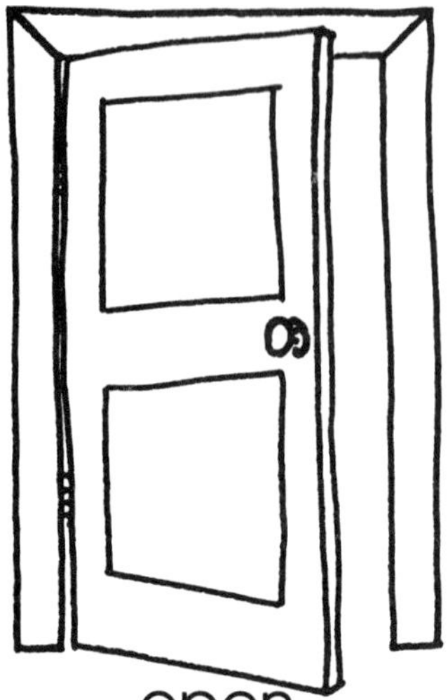

open

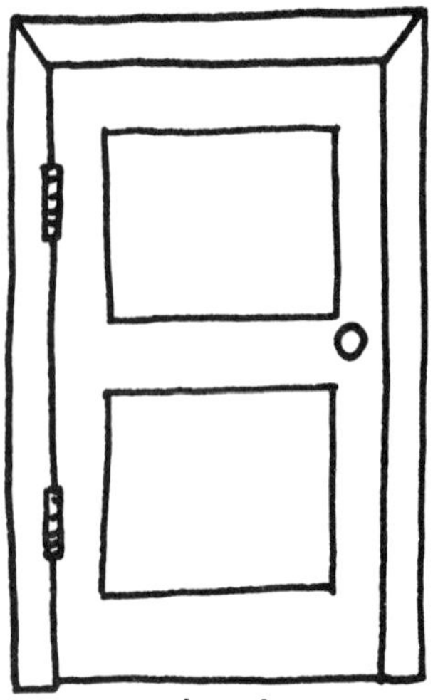

shut

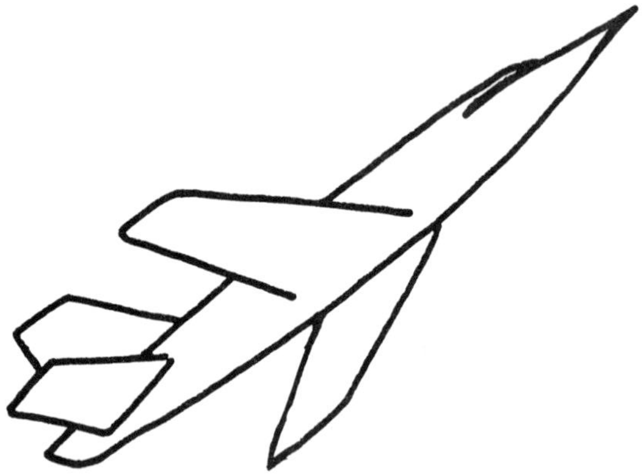

fast

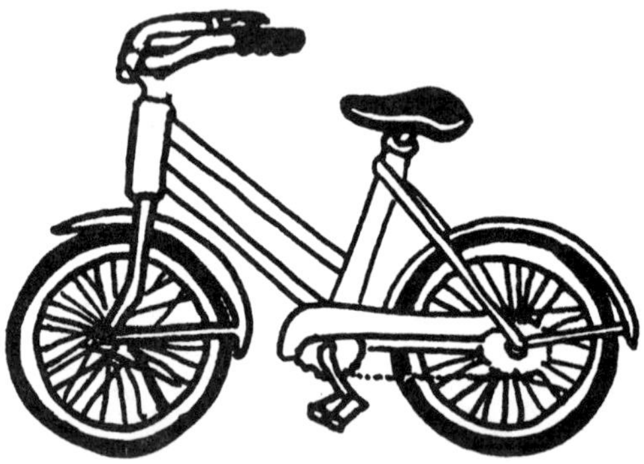

slow

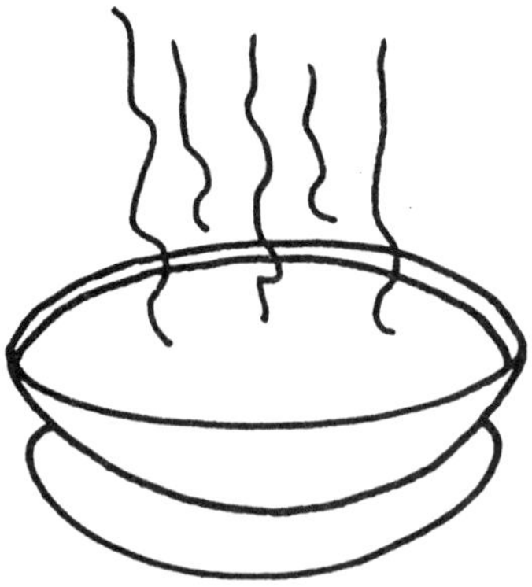

hot

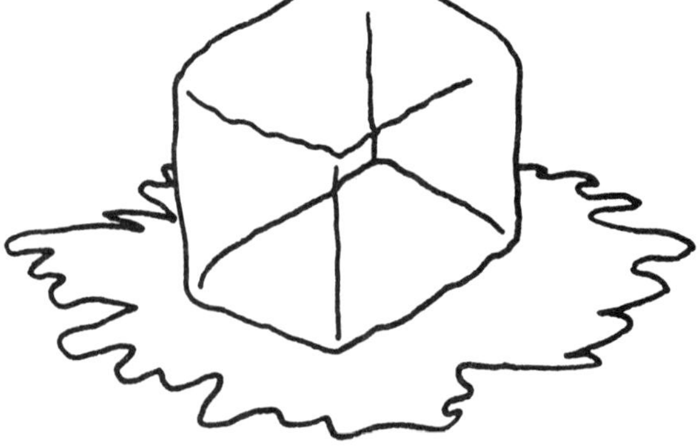

cold

OVER and UNDER

Materials: Flannel board
Cut-outs of several shapes, such as umbrella, apple, star, ball (page 29)
Ball
Box or bag

5. *Introduce concepts "over" and "under."* The ball is on the board. I will put the star over the ball. I will put the apple under the ball. Where is the star? Yes, it is over the ball. Where is the apple? The apple is under the ball.

   Remove cut-outs. I have put the apple on the board. *Place star over it.* Where have I put the star? *Move star under the apple.* Where is the star now? *Ask each child as objects are moved. Place one cut-out on board. Give each child a cut-out.* Put your cut-out on the board under the car. *Continue until each child has placed his cut-out. After all cut-outs are on the board, ask children questions.* Where did ________________ put her cut-out?

FAST and SLOW

Materials: Books
Pictures that illustrate "fast" and "slow"

6. *Place pictures illustrating "fast" and "slow" on the table.* This is a picture of something fast. Show a picture of something slow. Now, you choose a picture, and tell if the object is fast or slow.

OPEN and CLOSED

7. *Introduce concepts of "open" and "closed." Stand by door.* The door is open. *Close the door.* I have closed the door. *Open the door.* Is the door open or closed? Yes, the door is open. *Open and close door, calling children to tell whether it is open or closed*

   Place a book on the table. This book is closed. *Open the book.* Now, the book is open. ________________, is the book open or closed? *Open and close book calling all children to respond.*

NARROW and WIDE

Materials: Chairs
Strips of paper, some narrow, some wide
Objects that are narrow and wide, such as ribbon, cloth, wood
Objects that are thick and thin, such as pencils, crayons, books

8. *Introduce concepts of "narrow" and "wide." Place two chairs close together and two chairs much farther apart.* Let's play "Follow The Leader." We are going to go between each set of chairs, but we cannot touch the chairs. Be careful as you pass through. Follow me. *Lead children through both sets of chairs several times.*

   We passed through both sets of chairs. Let's look at the chairs. Was it easy to pass through both sets? No, it was not. *Point to chairs close together.* It was not easy to pass between these chairs. The space between these chairs is narrow. There is very little room. *Point to the chairs father apart.* These chairs were easier to pass through. The space between these chairs is wide. There is plenty of room. We can say something is narrow *(point to chairs close together),* or we can say something is wide *(point to chairs farther apart).*

9. *Put strips of paper on table. Mix them.* Look at these strips of paper. Some of the strips are narrow. *Hold up narrow strips.* Some of the strips are wide. *Hold up wide strips.*

   Let's put the narrow strips of paper over here and the wide strips over there. *Indicate places.* Choose a strip of paper, and tell if it is narrow or wide. Say: "This strip is narrow" or "This strip is wide." Then, put it in the correct place. *Call each child to choose strip, identify strip, and put strip in correct place.*

THICK and THIN

10. *Introduce concepts of "thick" and "thin," using objects. Point to books side by side. Then, point to thin book and say,* This book is thin. *Point to thick book and say:* This book is thick. *Point to thick crayon and say,* This crayon is bigger than this crayon. We say it is thick. *Then, point to objects and say:* This crayon is thin. Is this crayon thick or thin? Yes, it is thick. Is this book thick or thin? Yes, the book is thin. ___________________, point to a thick item. ___________________, point to a thin item. *Ask each child to respond.* Now, choose an object, and tell if it is thick or thin.

PROGRESS CHECK

Materials: Pictures of objects that illustrate these concepts – "clean" and "dirty," "old" and "new," "wet" and "dry," "hot" and "cold," "fast" and "slow"

Place pictures or objects on table by category ("old" and "new;" "dirty" and "clean;" "wet" and "dry;" "cold" and "hot," "fast" and "slow"). Select an object from the "old" and "new" category, and say: Tell if this is old or new.

Or: Choose a picture, and tell if the object is old or new. *Repeat activity, selecting picture or objects from each category.*

Scoring:

+	Identifies all concepts correctly
0	Fails to identify all concepts correctly

Readiness: Level E

Activity 3: Sentences

Objective: To use a sentence pattern with future tense

Materials: Large empty bag
Empty boxes and cans of foods or pictures of foods

1. *Ask each child to give name, using a complete sentence.* Now, please tell how you will get home from school this afternoon. Use a complete sentence. I will go first. I'll ride home from school in a car. ___________________, how will you get home from school? *Ask each child individually. If a child answers with only one word, such as "car," say:* You will ride in a car. Now say, "I will ride in a car."

2. Let's take a shopping trip. *Put a bag filled with empty boxes and cans or pictures of food items on table.* Let's pretend we will go to the grocery store. Select an item from the bag, and tell what you will buy at the store. I'll go first. *Choose an item from the bag, and tell the children:* I will buy some cereal. Now you try. *Give each child the opportunity to select and describe an item, using this pattern:* "I will buy ___________________." *If a child answers with only one word, such as "orange," say:* Yes, you will buy an orange. Now, you say, "I will buy an orange."

Materials: Large bag
Toys or pictures of toys

3. Today, we will talk about what you will do when you get home from school. I'll go first. I will cook dinner for my family when I get home from school. ___________________, what will you do when you get home from school? *If a child answers with only one word, such as "eat," say:* You will eat when you get home from school. Now say: "I will eat when I get home from school."

4. Let's take a shopping trip. We are going to the toy store. *Put a bag filled with toys or pictures on the table.* Let's pretend we will go to the toy store. Select an item from the bag, and tell what you will buy at the store. I'll go first. *Choose item from bag, and show children.* I will buy a doll. Now, you try.

   Ask each child to select and describe item, using pattern. I will buy ___________________.
   If a child answers with one word say: Yes, you will buy a truck. Now say, "I will buy a truck."

Toys

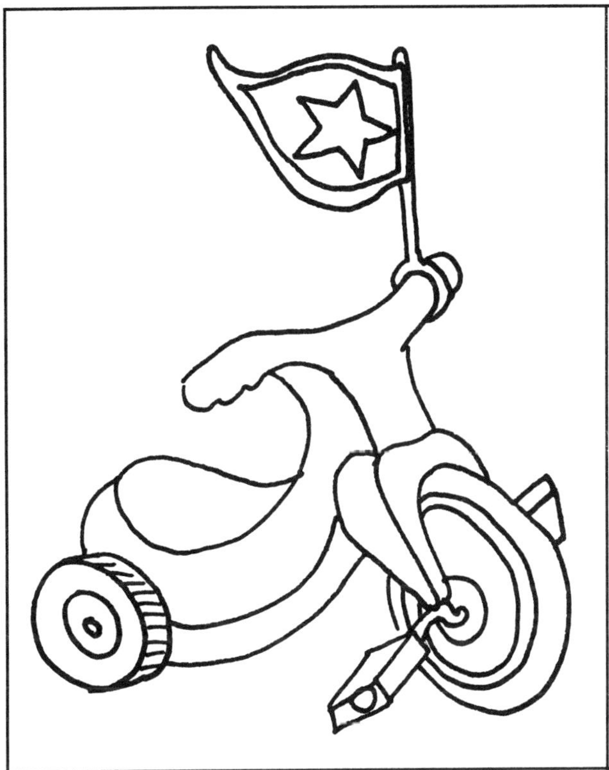
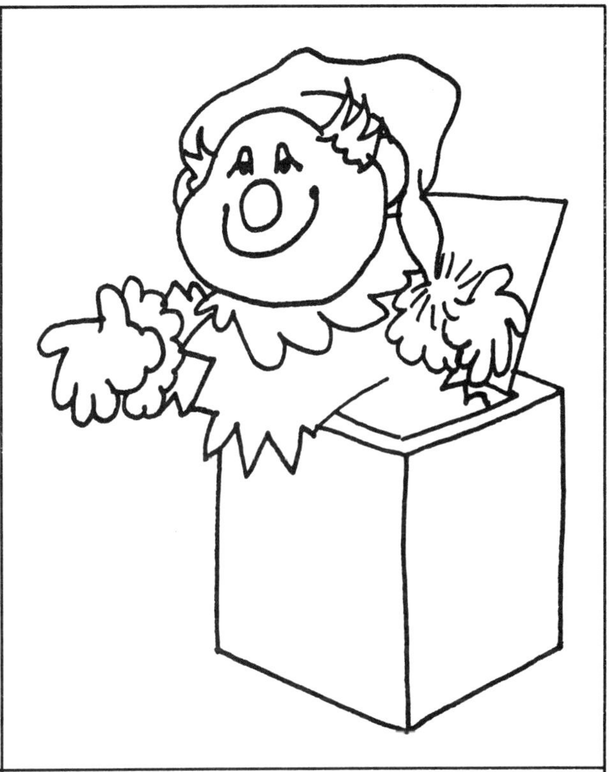
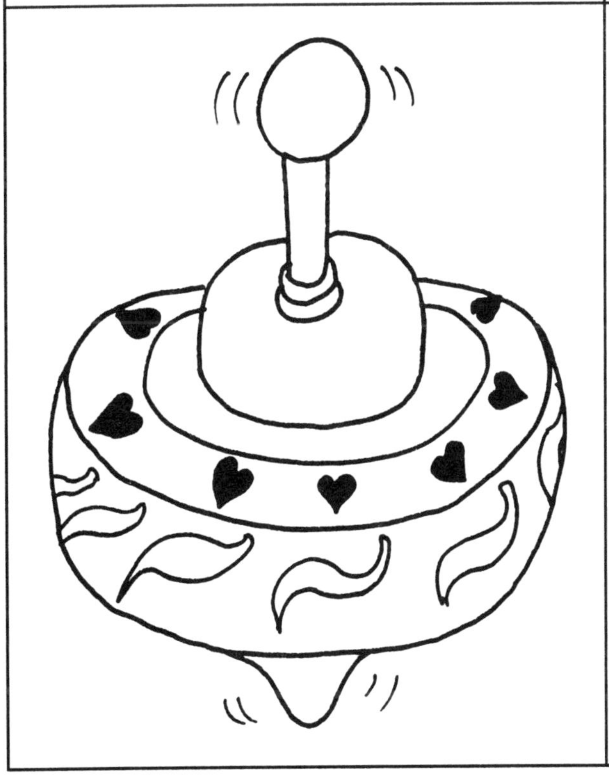
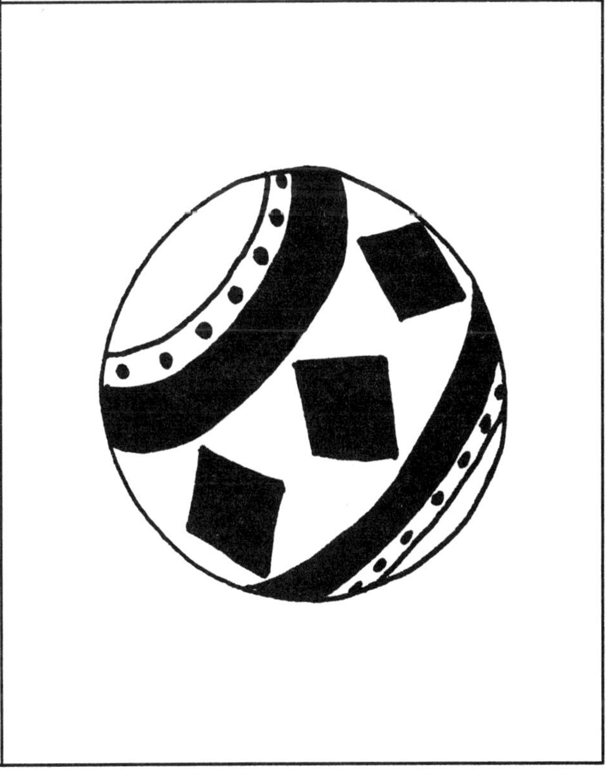

Materials: Flannel board
Felt cut-outs of familiar objects, such as apple, star (page 29)
Yarn

5. *Place yarn on flannel board in the shape of a circle. Show cut-out of apple. Say*: I will put the apple in the circle. Place the apple in the circle.

   Did I place the apple where I told you I would put it? Yes. Now, I will give each of you an object to place on the flannel board. You may place your object in the circle, under the circle, on top of the circle, beside the circle, any place as long as you put it on the flannel board. But, before you place your object, you must tell where you are going to put it. Use a complete sentence.

Materials: Paper stars
Masking tape

6. *Place folded tape on the back of paper stars so the stars will stick to objects. Show the stars to the children. Say:* I want you to put the star somewhere on your body. But first, you must tell where you will put your star. Watch me. I will put my star on my arm. *Put the star on your arm. Ask a child:*

   ____________________, where will you put your star?

   Model sentences, such as: "I will put the star on my arm."

7. I have a poem to share today. *Teach:*

   Star light, star bright,
   First star I see tonight.
   I wish I may,
   I wish I might
   Have the wish I wish tonight.

   When you see the first star at night, you can make a wish. Let's pretend it is night. We look at the sky, and see the first star. What will you wish for? I'll go first. I'll wish for____________________ when I see the star.

Girl and Clothes

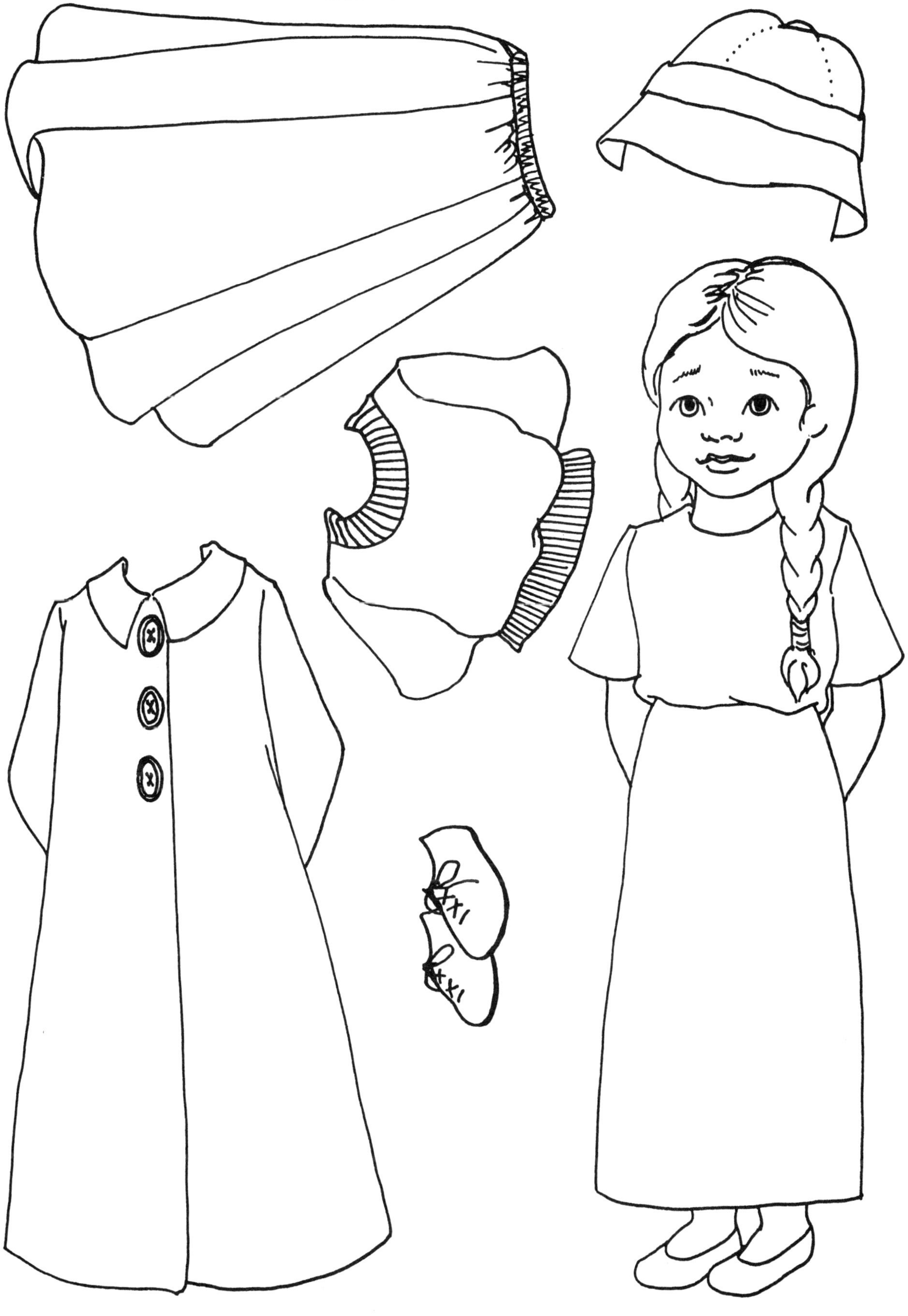

Materials: Flannel board
Felt cut-outs of body
Felt cut-outs of clothing

8. *Put the body on the flannel board. Say:* This is Cindy. Cindy is getting ready to go to school, but she can't decide what to wear. Let's help Cindy by choosing clothes for her to wear to school. Please choose an article of clothing to put on Cindy, and tell what you chose.

Allow each child the opportunity to select an item of clothing, then say, "I will put the ____________________ on Cindy."

Now, Cindy has come home from school. She is ready for a nap. Let's help by removing the clothes. ____________________, please take an article of clothing off Cindy, but tell what you are going to do first by saying: "I will take the ____________________ off Cindy."

Materials: Large bag
Toys

9. *Put the materials on the table. Say:*

Let's play a game called "Bag It." You'll play this game with a buddy. I will show you how to play the game with ____________________. ____________________, sit with me. ____________________, choose a toy to put in the bag. Which toy will you put in the bag?

Encourage use of sentences.

I will put the ____________________ in the bag. Now, I will take ____________________'s toy out of the bag, but first, I will tell you what I will do with the toy. I'll play with the doll that ____________________ put in the bag.

Pair children to play the game. Supervise them, encouraging responses.

10. I want you to tell what you will do when you get home from school this afternoon. Use a complete sentence. I'll go first. I will bake a cake when I get home from school today. ____________________, what will you do when you get home from school today?

You will eat when you get home from school. Now say: "I will eat when I get home from school."

PROGRESS CHECK

Materials: None

Ask each child four questions. If a child fails to answer the first question with a complete sentence using future tense, prompt one time. Give no additional prompts. Ask questions, such as:

What will you do when you get home tonight?
How will you come to school tomorrow?
What will you eat tonight?
What will you have for breakfast tomorrow morning?
What will you do during recess this afternoon?

Scoring:

+	Answers four questions, using complete sentences without prompts
0	Fails to answer four questions, using complete sentences without prompts

Readiness: Level E

Activity 4: Sequencing

Objective: To place objects in sequence and explain how this was done

Materials: Small cup
Small blocks
Clay

1. *Perform a routine familiar to the children. Say:* Watch me carefully. *Get a cup. Put water in it. Ask:* What did I do first? What did I do next? What did I do last?

2. *Place small blocks on table. Say:* Watch me carefully. *Stack the blocks on top of each other until they fall. Ask*: What did I do first? What did I do next? What did I do last?

3. *Build a snowman with clay by making three balls (one large, one medium, one small) and stacking them on top of each other. Make eyes, nose, and mouth in the head. Ask:* What did I do first? What did I do next? What did I do last?

Materials: Toys
Illustrated book of nursery rhymes

4. *Give children simple tasks to do, such as:* ____________________, please walk to my desk, get a pencil, and bring it to me. *When task is completed, ask:* What did you do first? What did you do next? What did you do last? *Give each child the opportunity to participate by giving each child different directions to follow. Discuss.*

Materials: Three sets of two pictures each that can be sequenced

5. *Introduce each set of pictures. Show the first picture, and ask children to discuss it in detail. Prompt whenever necessary; ask questions to obtain more information. Then, show the second picture in series, and ask children to describe it, as above.*

   Display each set of pictures. Ask: What do you think happened before the first picture? What do you think happened after the last picture? *Continue for each set of pictures, giving each child ample opportunity to participate.*

Sequencing Pictures: Two Scenes

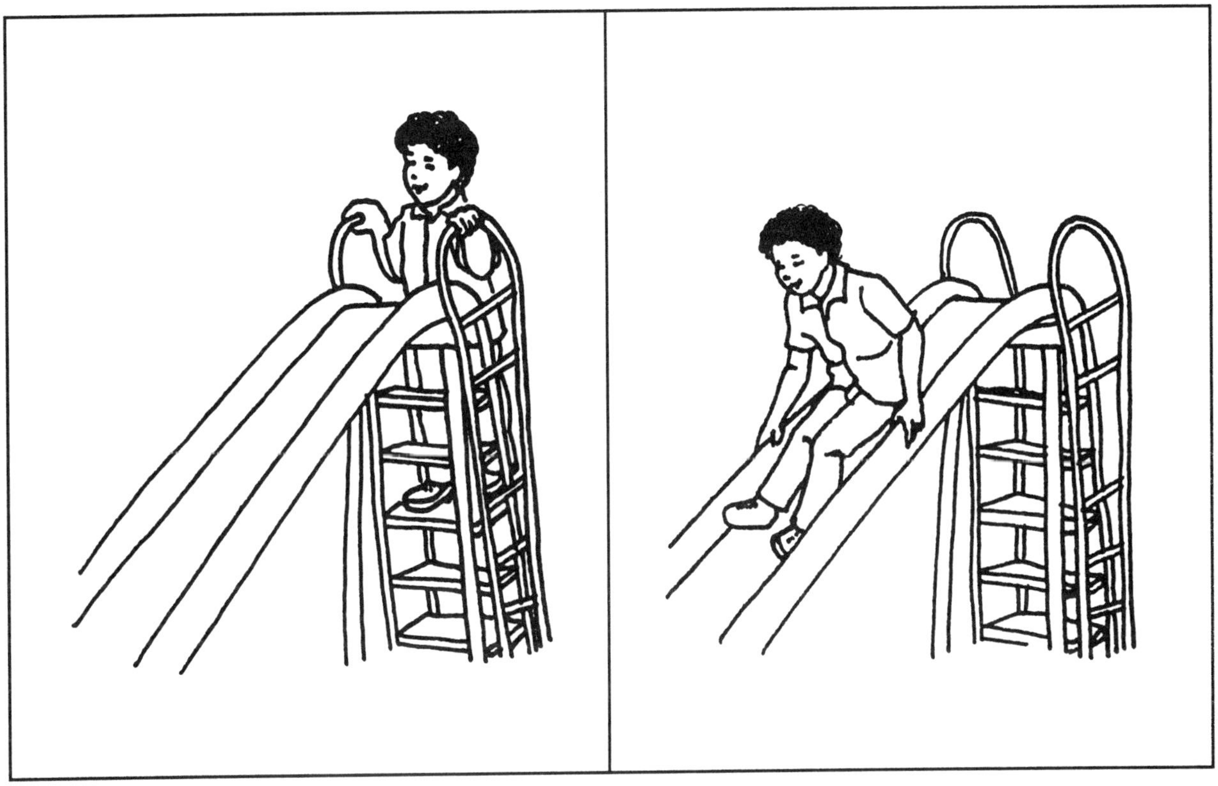

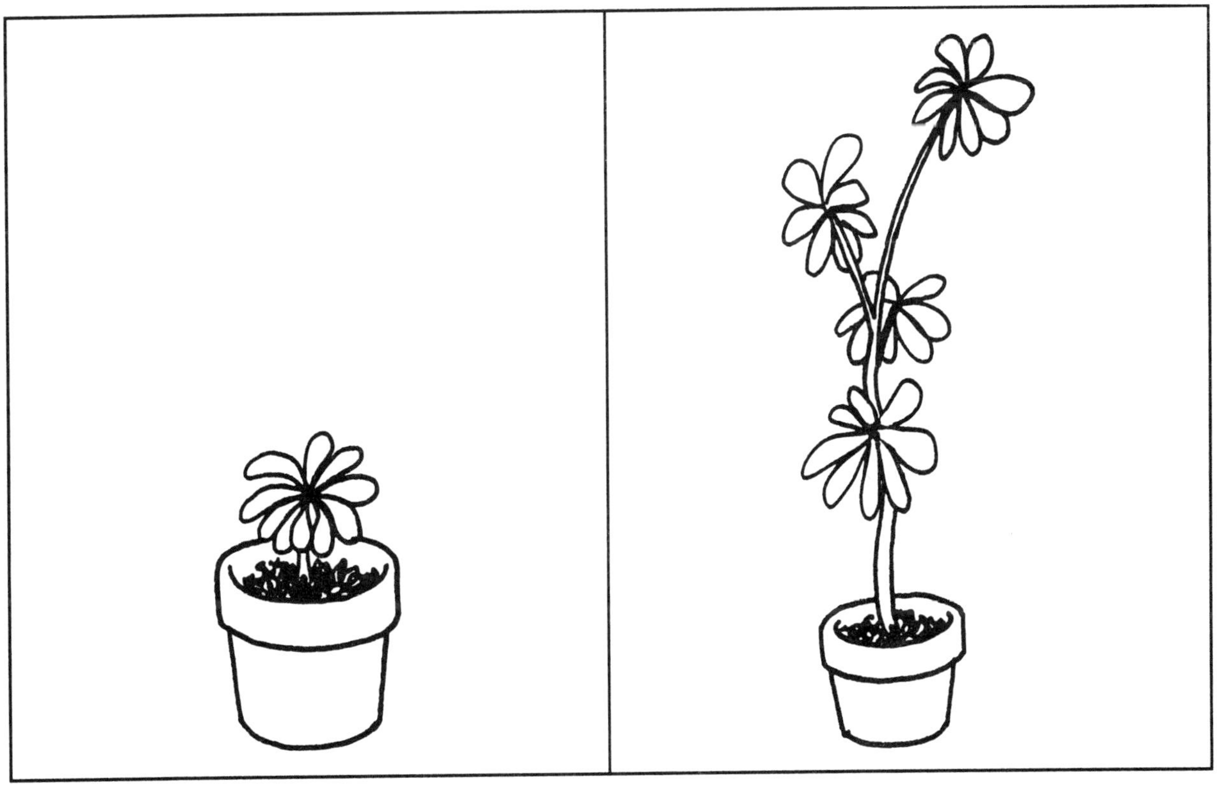

Sequencing Pictures: Two Scenes

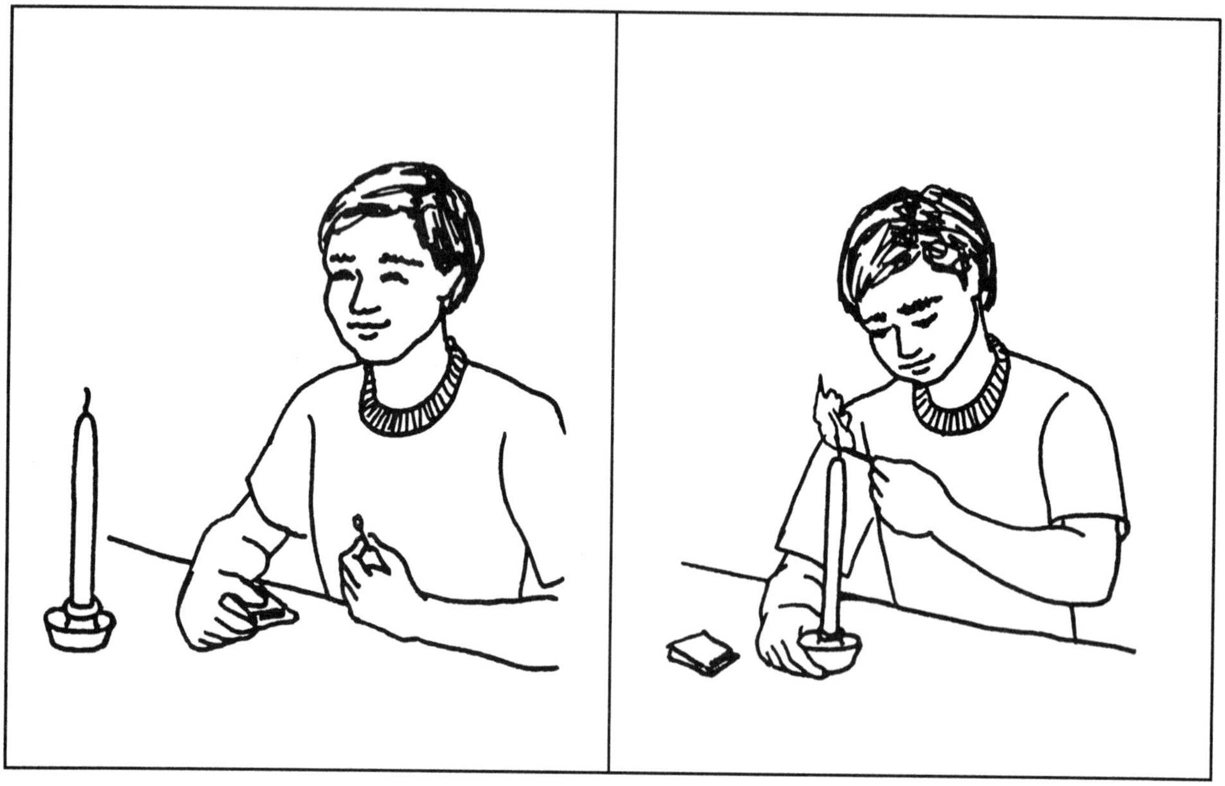

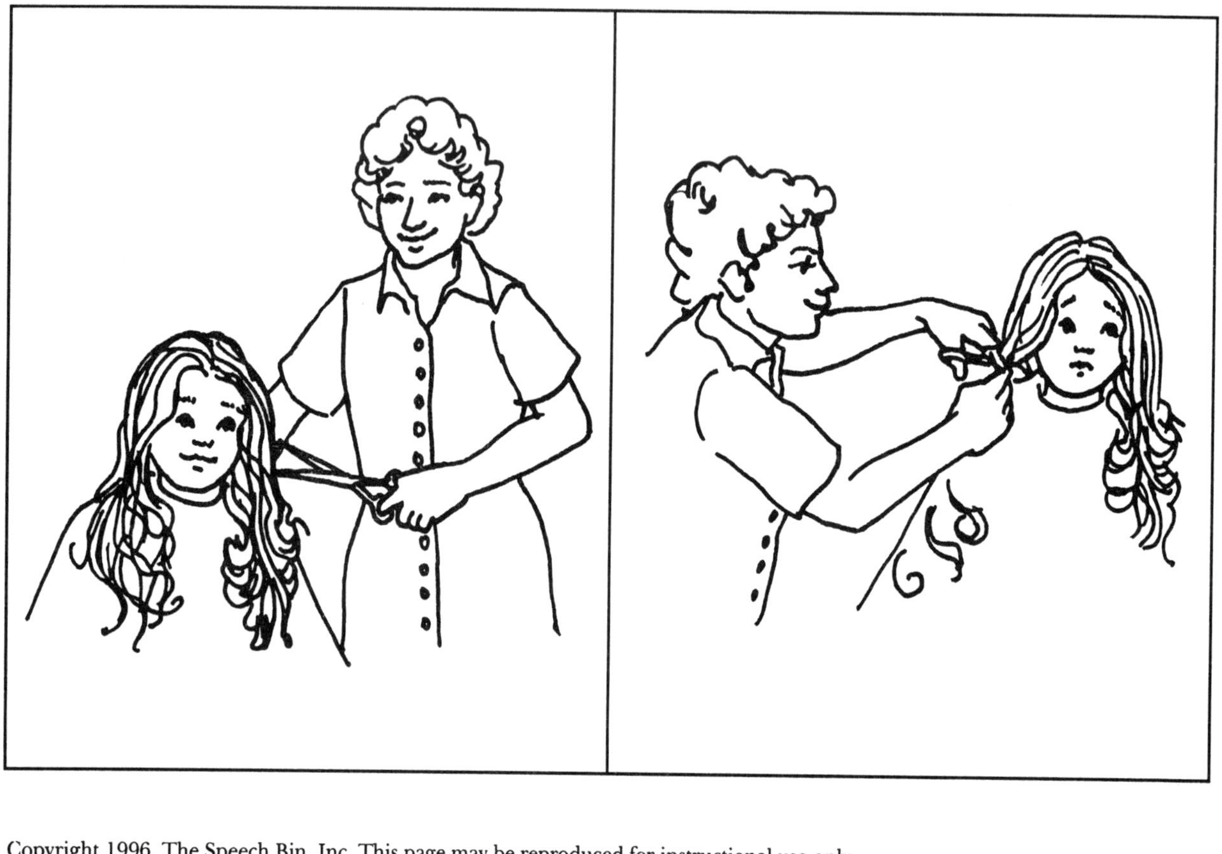

6. When I got up this morning, first, I washed my face. Next, I brushed my teeth. Last, I put on my clothes. Tell me what you did first, next, and last this morning. *Encourage use of complete sentences that include the words "first," "next," and "last."*

Materials: Three sets of three pictures each that can be sequenced

7. *Display a set of pictures. Show pictures to the children in sequence. Point to the first picture. Ask:* What is happening in this picture? *Repeat for the remaining two pictures. When completed, give first picture in the sequence to a child. Ask:* Who has the picture that comes first? Show us the picture, and tell us about it. *Continue for "next" and "last" pictures. Then scramble the pictures and give them to a child to put in order. Ask a child to tell what is happening in the pictures, using the words "first," "next," and "last."*

8. *Display a set of pictures for the children. Show them the middle picture of each set first. Point to the middle picture. Ask:* What is happening in this picture? *Give a child the other two pictures in the same set. Ask:* Which picture comes first? Put that picture on the table. Which picture comes last? Put that picture last on the table. Now, tell about all three pictures in the order in which they happened. *Continue with other sets of pictures, giving each child an opportunity to participate.*

Materials: Three sets of four pictures each that can be sequenced

9. *Introduce each set of pictures. Show the first picture, and ask children to describe it. Prompt when necessary. Ask questions to obtain more information. Then, show second picture in the series, and ask children to describe it, using the same procedure. Continue for the remaining two pictures in each set. After introducing each set, ask individual children to tell a story about the pictures, in order. Allow each child to participate individually, giving each one an opportunity.*

Sequencing Pictures: Four Scenes

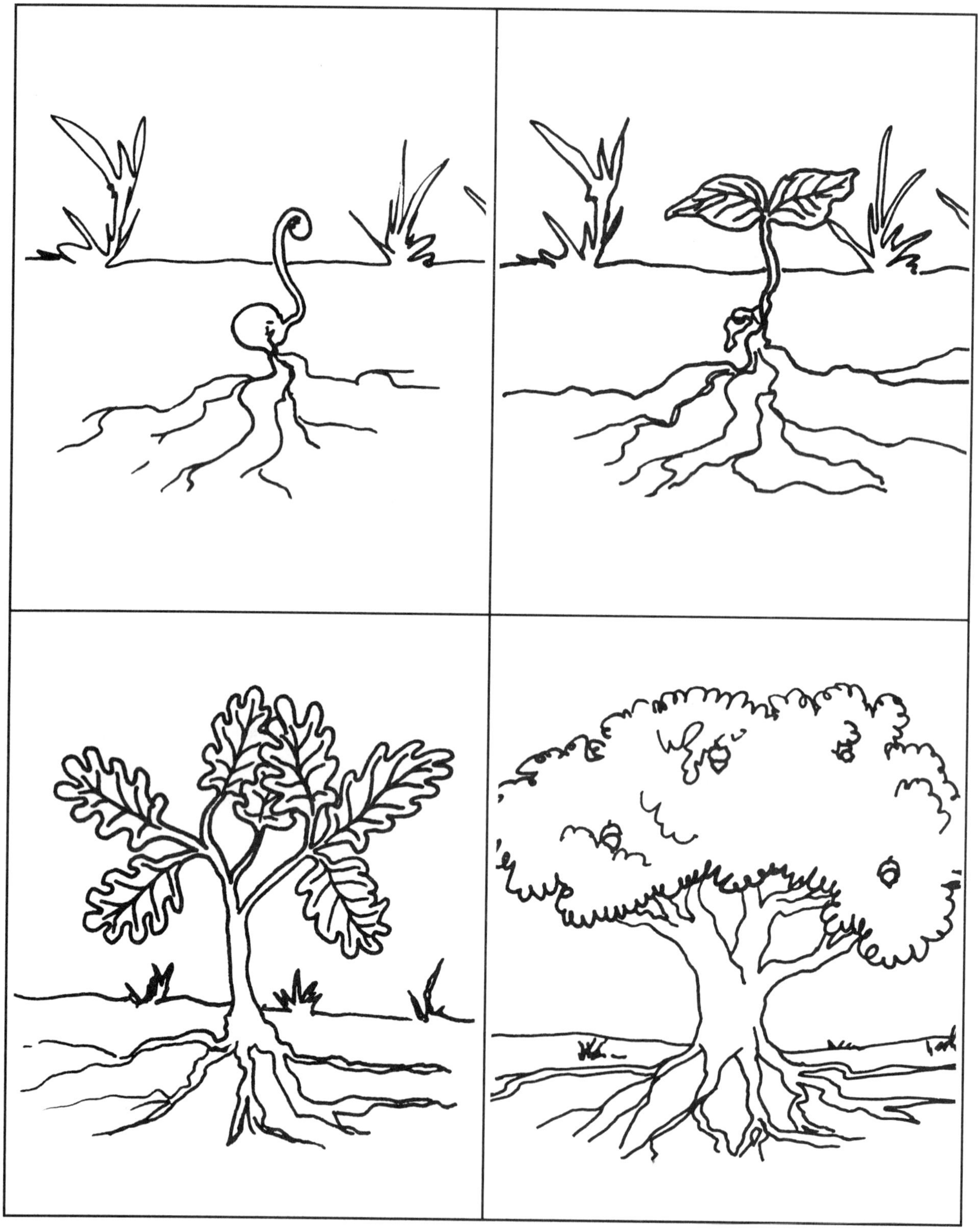

Sequencing Pictures: Four Scenes

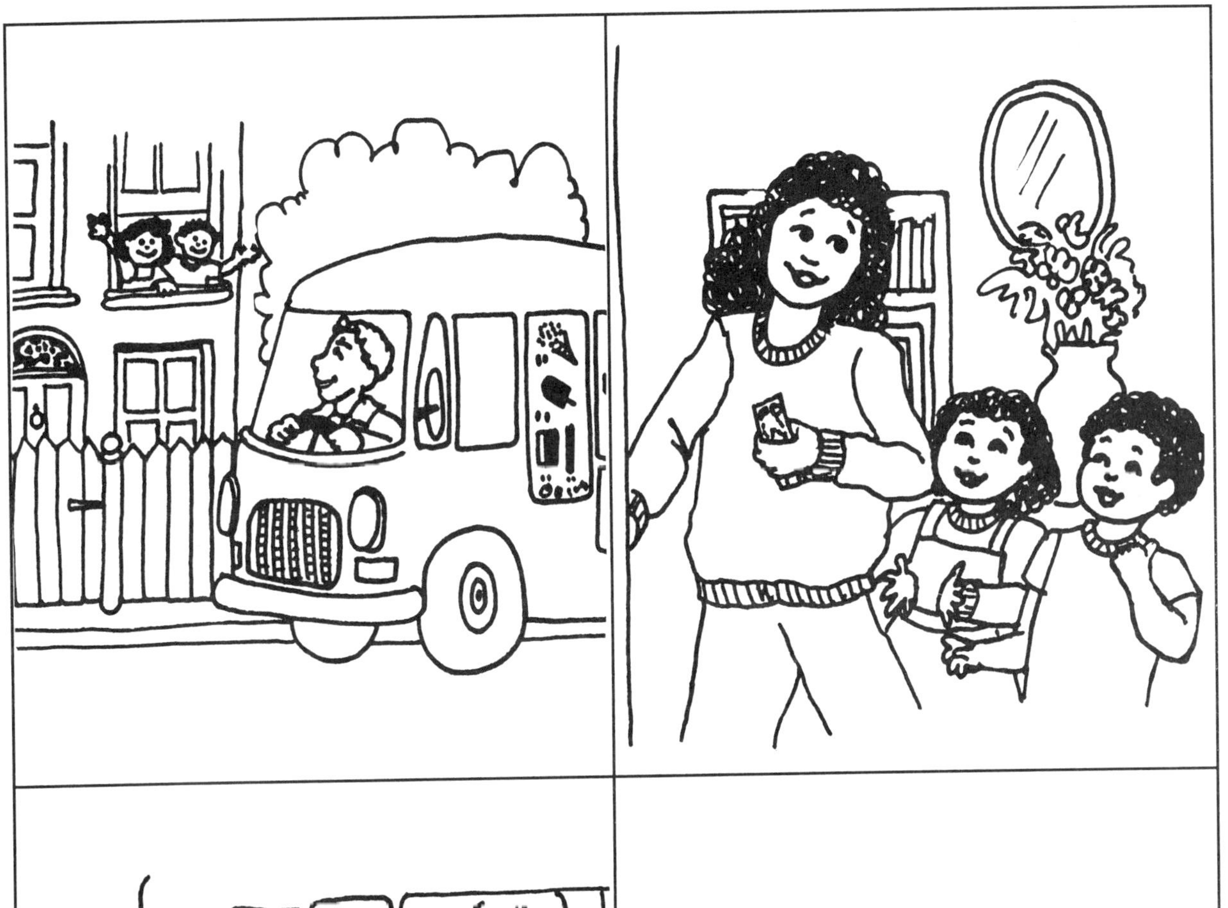

Sequencing Pictures: Four Scenes

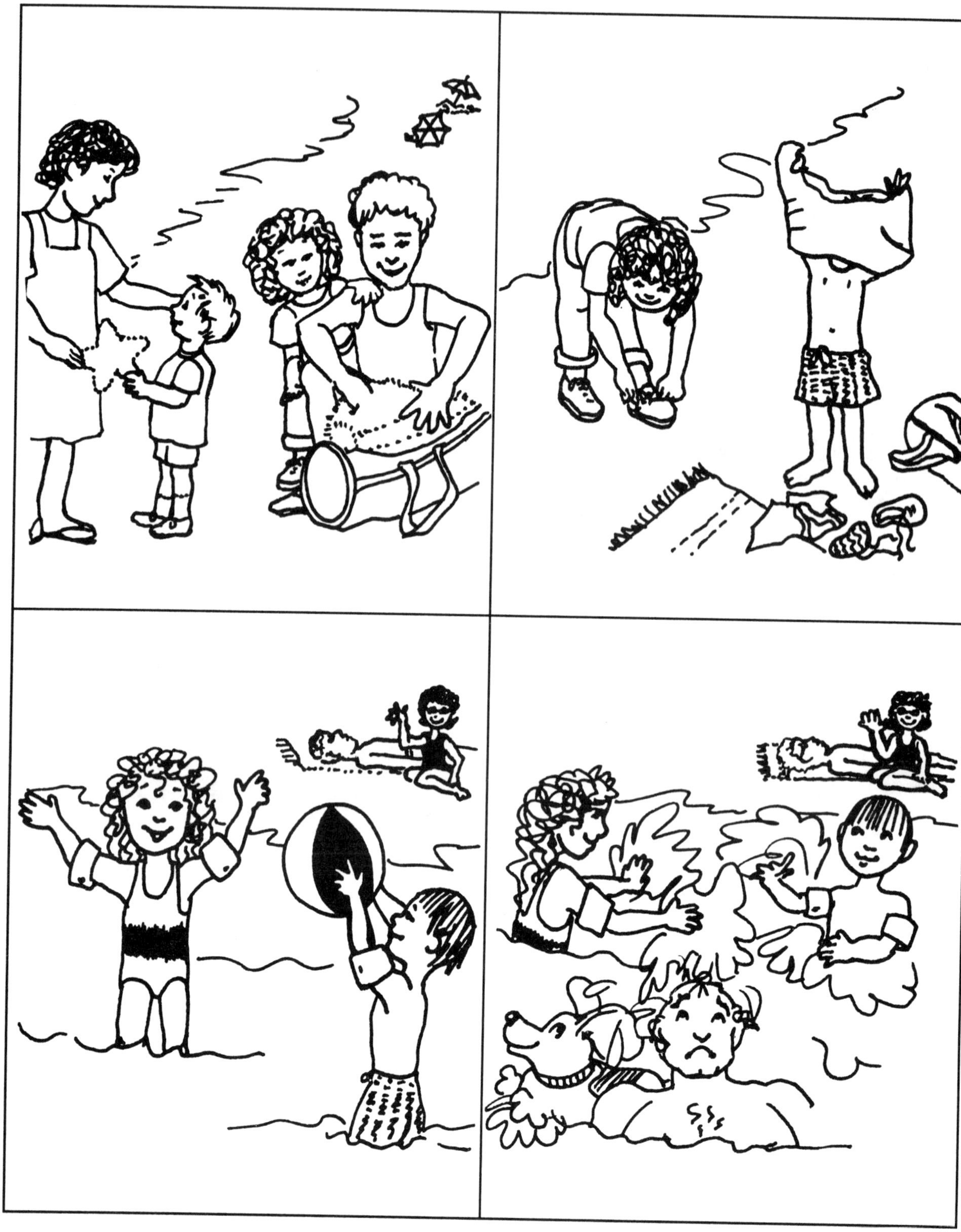

PROGRESS CHECK

Materials: Sets of four sequence pictures (previously used)

Display set of pictures, not in correct order. Ask child to put them in order, then tell about them. If necessary, say: What happened first? What happened next? *Give no more than one prompt. Observe.*

Scoring:

+	Sequences pictures correctly and tells story about them, using complete sentences (requiring no more than one prompt)
0	Fails to sequence pictures correctly and tell story about them, using complete sentences, with no more than two prompts)

Sequencing Pictures: Three Scenes

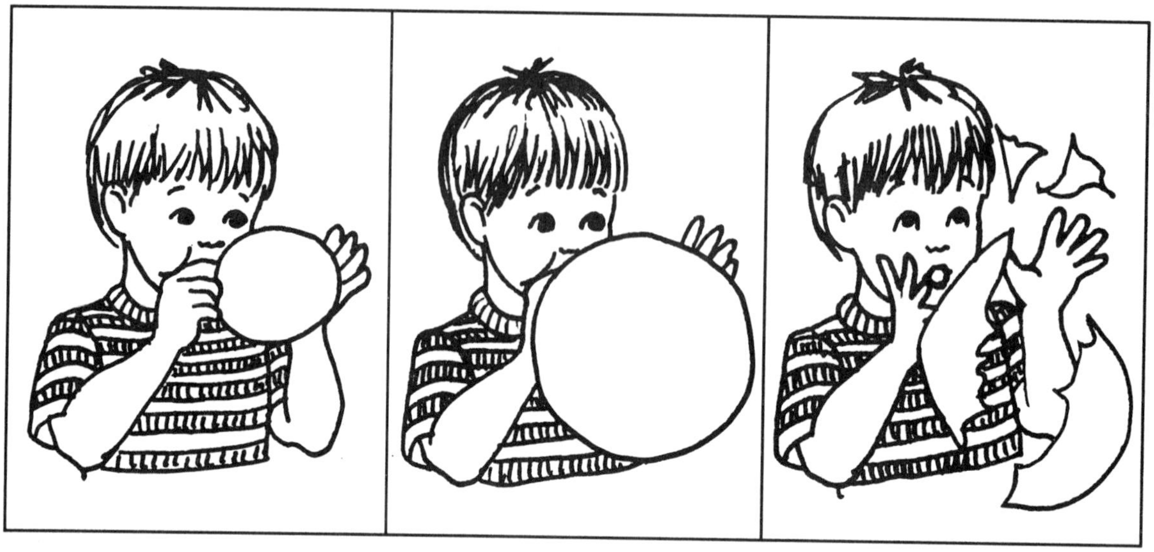

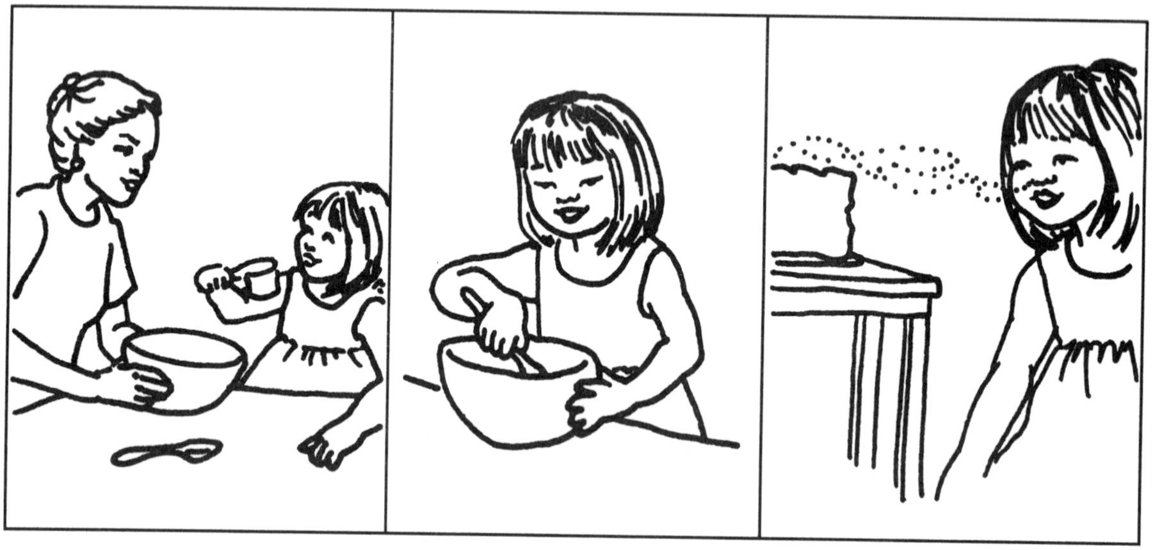

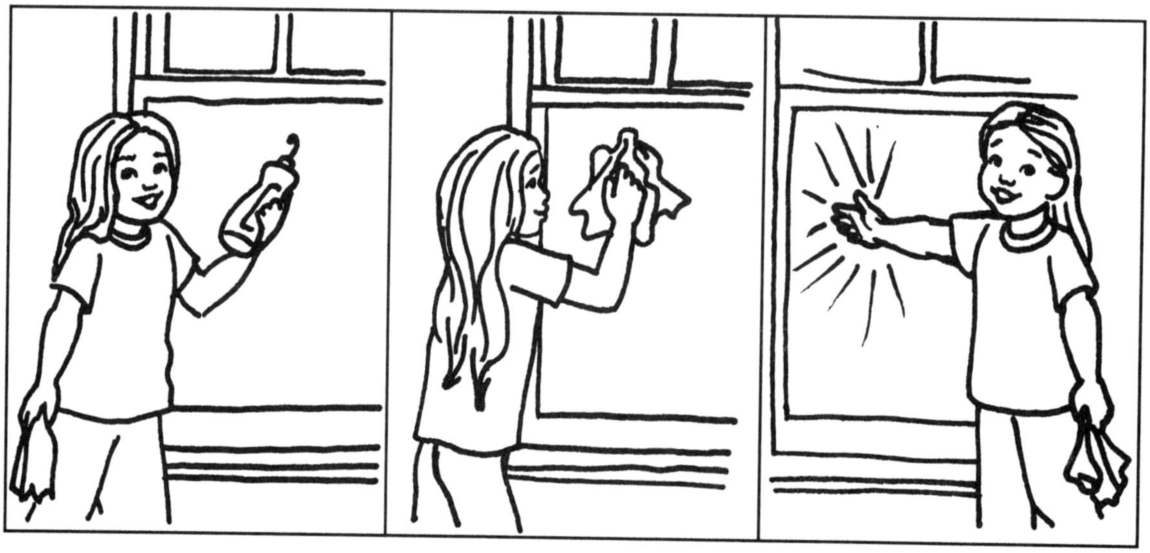

Sequencing Pictures: Three and Four Scenes

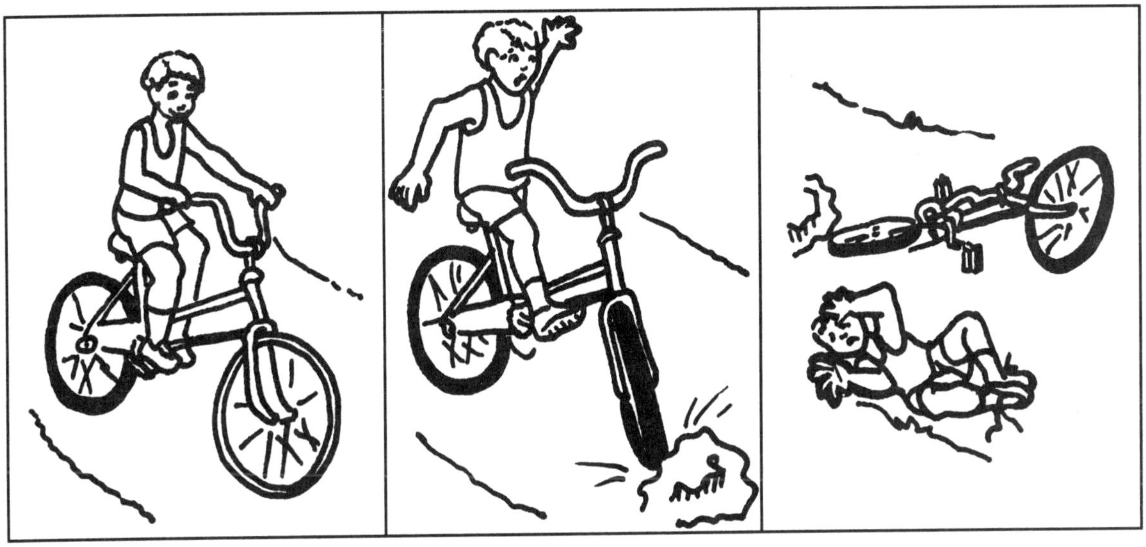

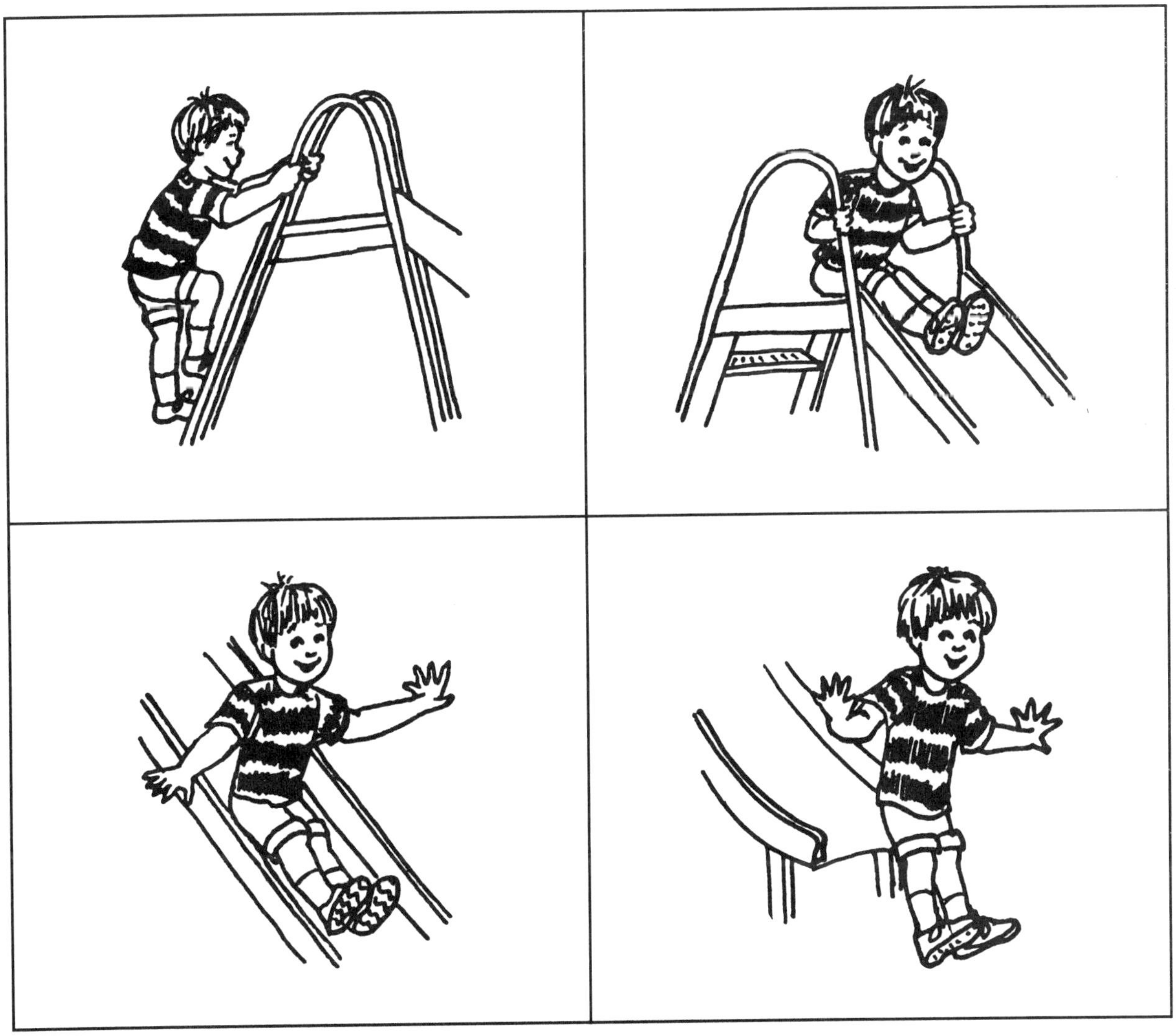

Readiness: Level E

Activity 5: Rhyming Words

Objective: To identify rhyming words

Materials: Nursery rhymes

1. I have a rhyme to share. Listen very carefully. *Repeat the first two lines of a nursery rhyme, such as "Jack and Jill." Emphasize the words that rhyme (example: "Jill" and "hill"). Say:* In this rhyme "Jill" and "hill" are two words that sound like each other. "Jill" and "hill" are called rhyming words because they have the same ending sounds. Now, you say them with me, and listen to their sounds. Jill...hill. Again. Jill...hill. Now, let's repeat the rhyme *(emphasize italicized words):*

   Jack and *Jill*
   Went up the *hill...*

   Continue with the first two lines of other nursery rhymes, emphasizing the rhyming words and asking children to repeat each rhyming pair.

Materials: Pairs of objects or pictures that rhyme (such as "sock" and "lock," "book" and "hook," "frog" and "log," "pan" and "fan," and "cat" and "hat")
Large bag

2. I have a rhyme to share. Listen very carefully, *Repeat the first two lines of a rhyme, such as "Little Jack Horner." Emphasize the words that rhyme ("Horner" and "corner"). Say:* In this rhyme "Horner" and "corner" are two words that sound like each other "Horner" and "corner" are called rhyming words because they have the same ending sounds. Now, you say them with me, and listen to their sounds. Horner...corner. Again. Horner...corner. Now, let's repeat the rhyme *(emphasize italicized words):*

   Little Jack *Horner*
   Sat in a *corner...*

   Continue with the first two lines of other nursery rhymes, emphasizing the rhyming words and asking children to repeat each rhyming pair.

3. *Display the objects or pictures. Say:* I have some objects (or pictures of objects) that rhyme. *Introduce each pair of objects; name them and emphasize the rhyming sounds. Ask children to repeat the names. Say:* Look at the "sock" and the "lock." Sock and lock rhyme. They both have the "ock" sound at the end. Let's say those two words. Listen to how they rhyme. Ready? Sock...lock. *Continue in the same way with other rhyming pairs.*

Picture Pairs

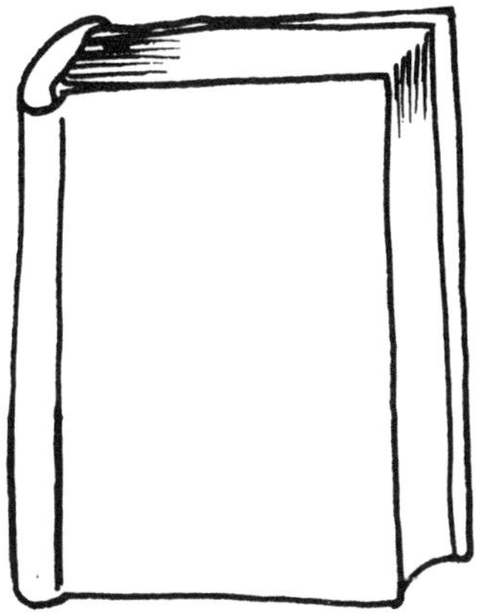

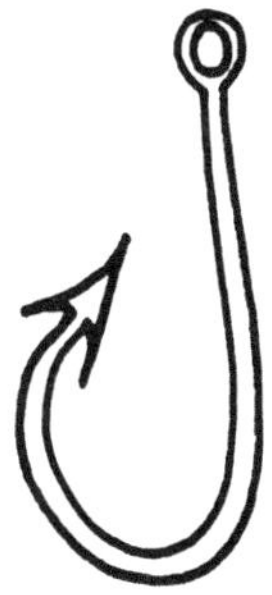

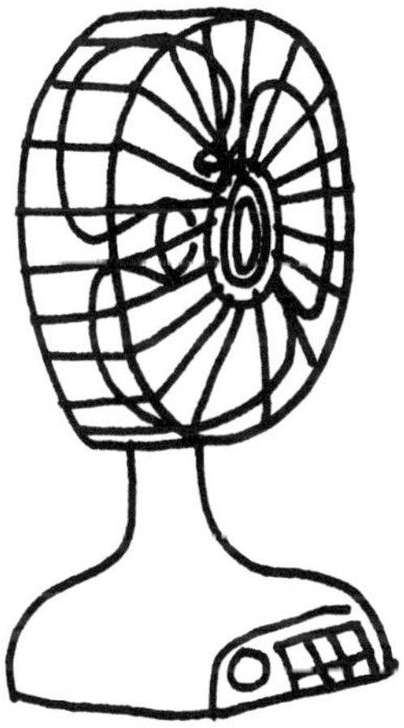

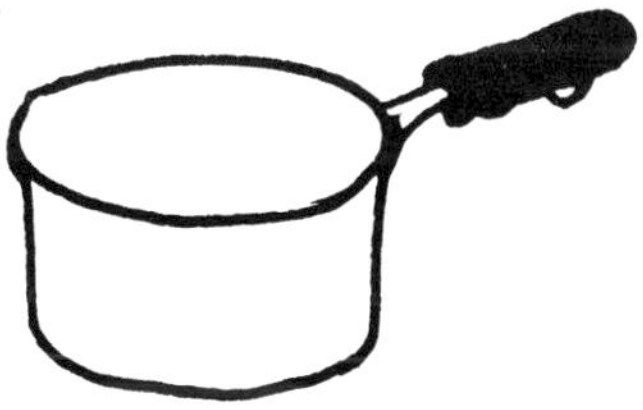

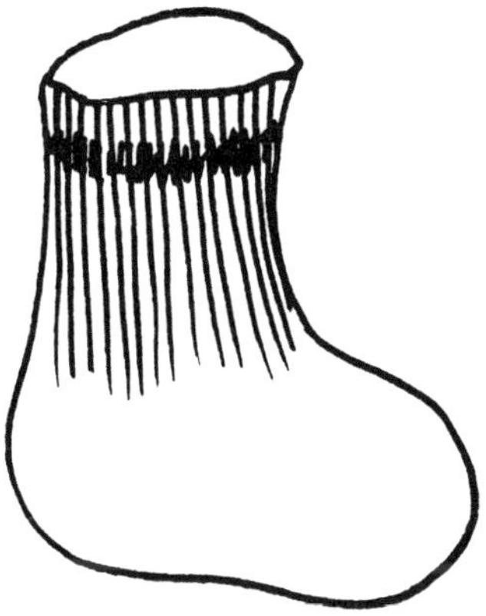

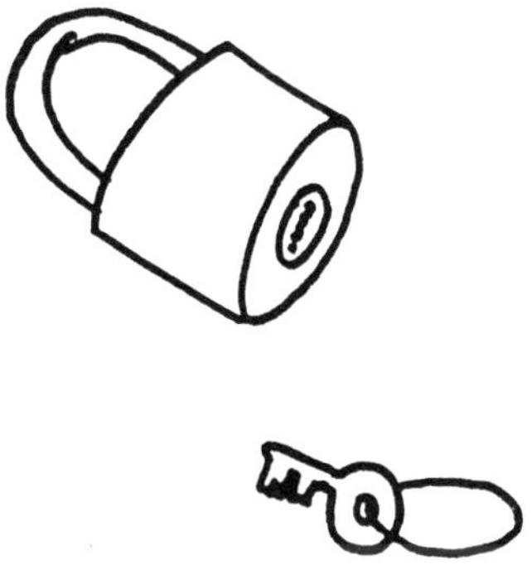

Picture Pairs

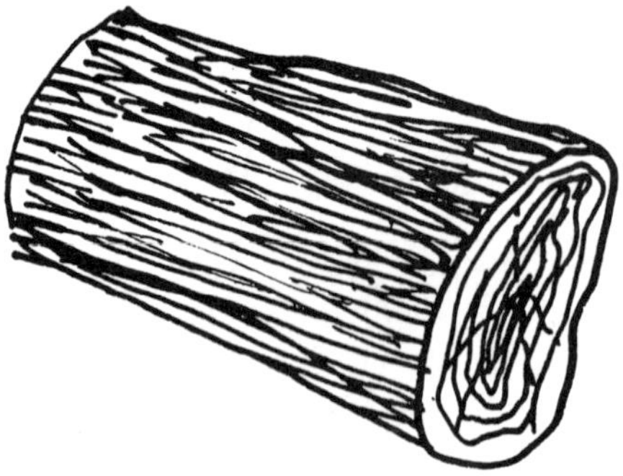

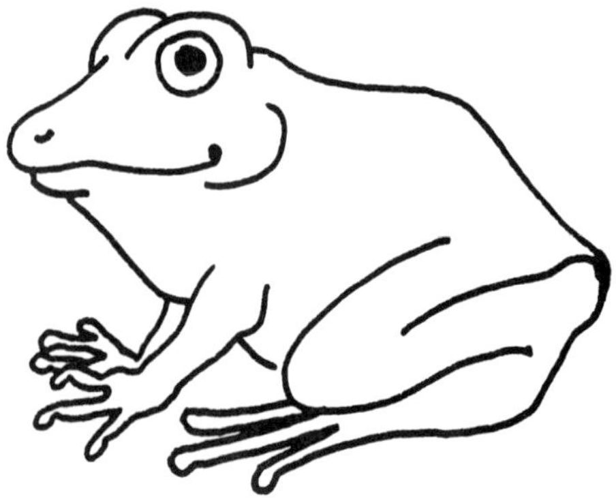

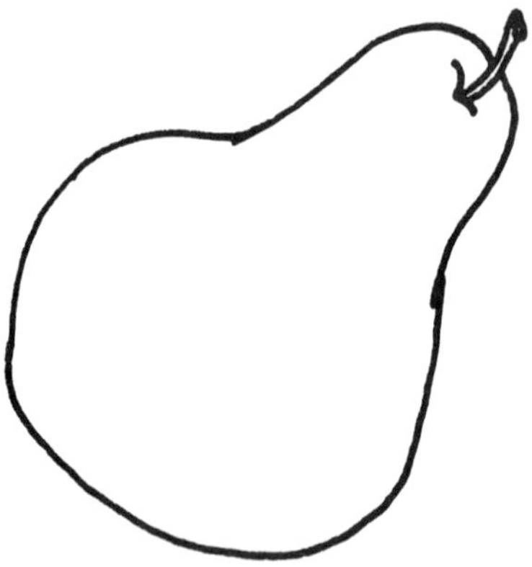

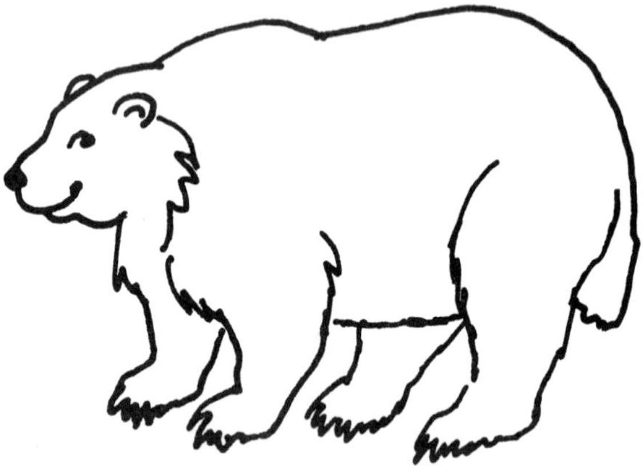

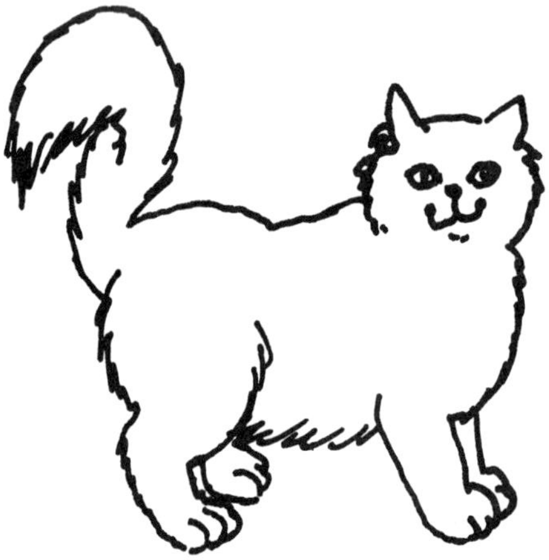

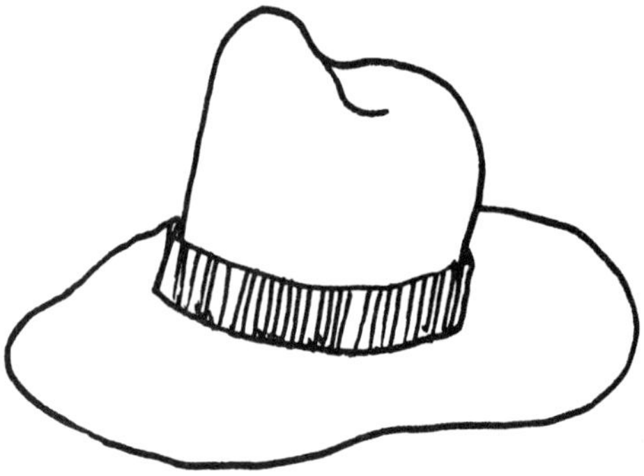

Picture Pairs

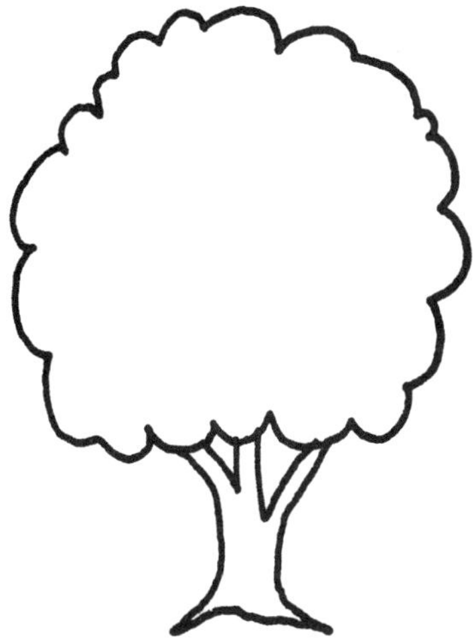

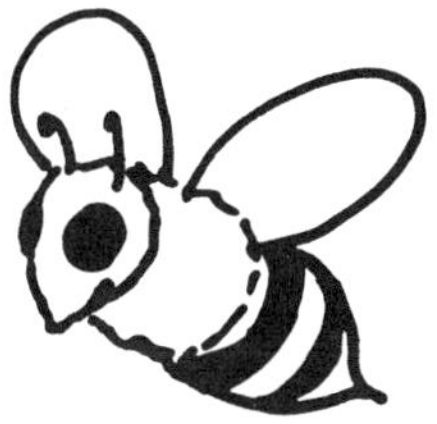

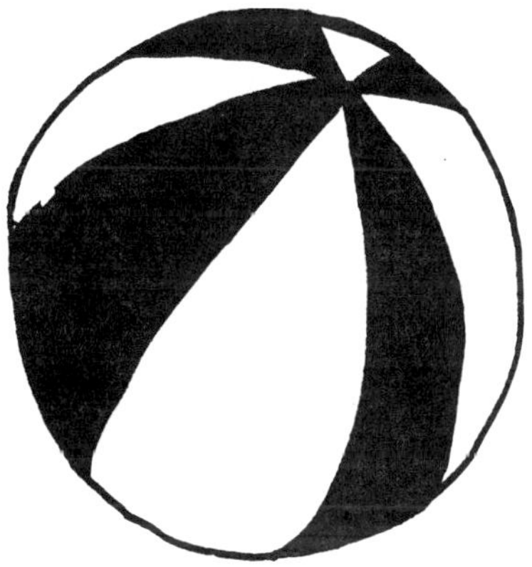

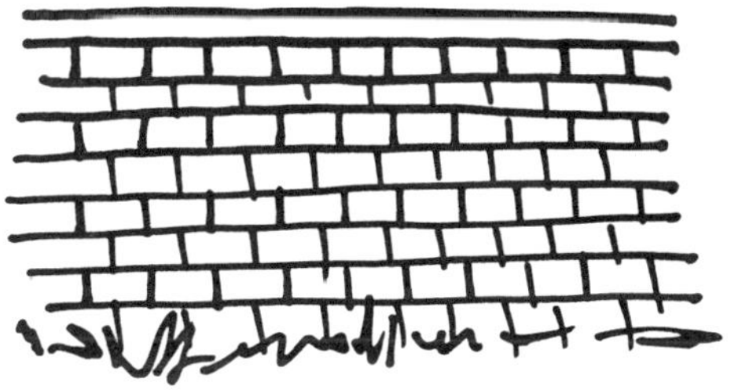

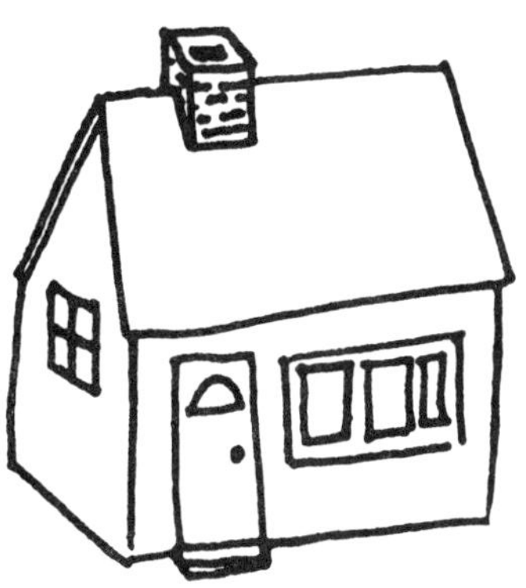

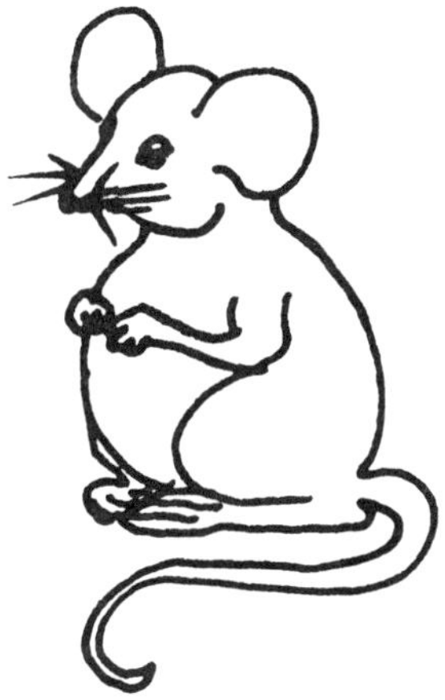

Picture Pairs

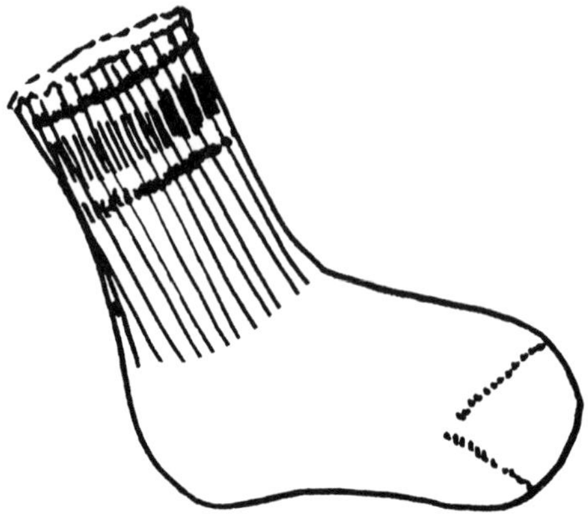

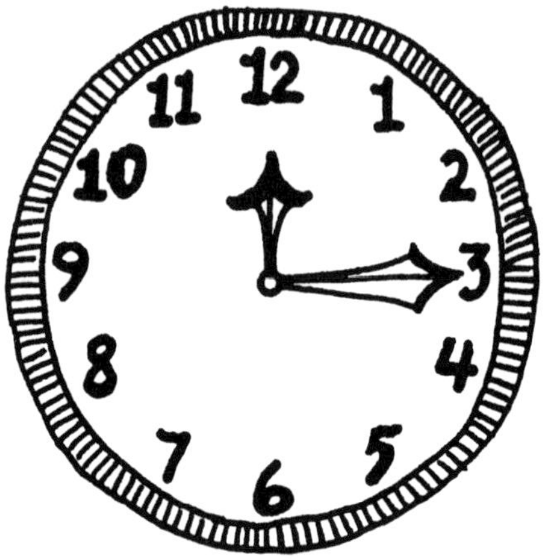

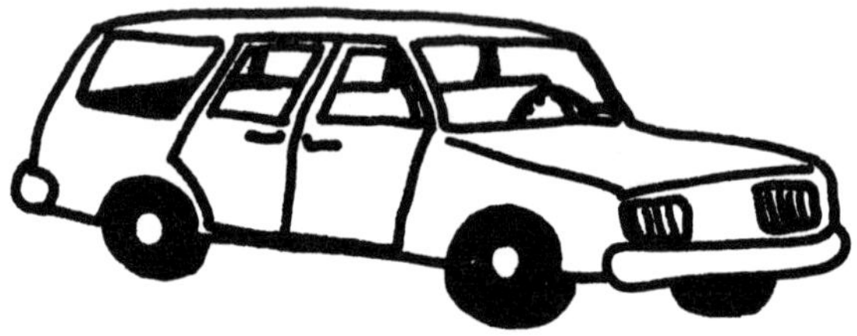

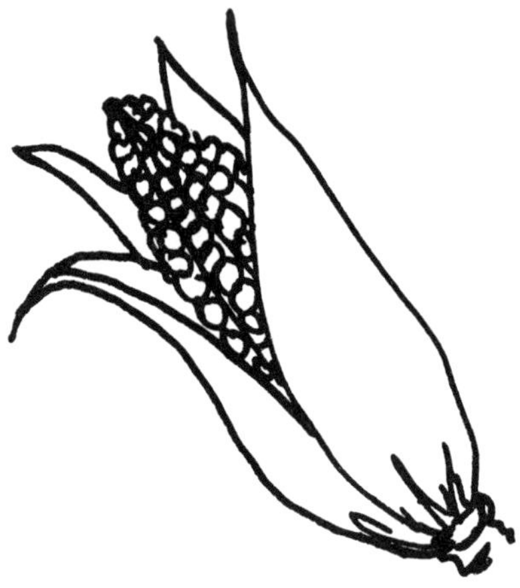

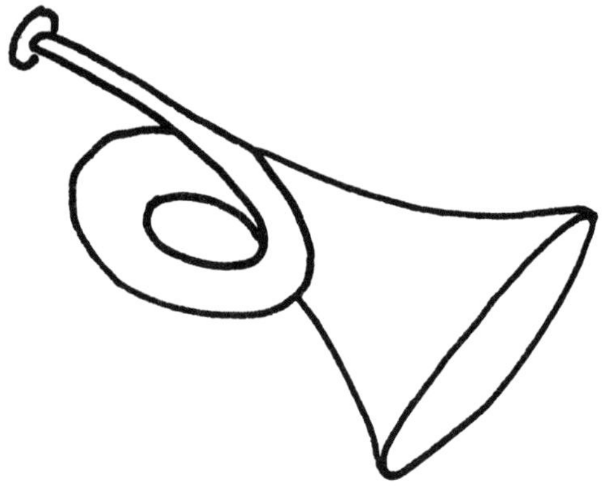

4. Let's play a game called "Rhyming Pairs." *Put one object (or picture) of each rhyming pair in a bag, and display the other on the table in front of the children. Say:* Choose an object (or picture) from the bag. Tell us its name. Then, find the object on the table that has a rhyming name. Say that name. Put the two objects that rhyme together. Ready? *Ask each child to select an object from the bag, locate its rhyming object, and name them.*

5. I have a rhyme to share. Listen very carefully. *Repeat the first two lines of a rhyme, such as "Little Miss Muffet." Emphasize the words that rhyme ("Muffet" and "tuffet"). Say:* In this rhyme "Muffet" and "tuffet" are two words that sound like each other. "Muffet" and "tuffet" are called rhyming words because they have the same ending sounds. Now, you say them with me, and listen to their sounds. Muffet...tuffet. Again. Muffet...tuffet. Now, let's repeat the rhyme *(emphasize italicized words):*

    Little Miss *Muffet*
    Sat on a *tuffet...*

6. Listen carefully as I say two words that rhyme: "bat"..."cat." Again: "bat"..."cat." Both "bat" and "cat" have the "at" sound at the end. Now, you say them. Ready? Say: bat...cat. Again: bat...cat. Can you think of something we wear on our heads that rhymes with "bat" and "cat?" Yes, "hat" rhymes with "bat" and "cat." Let's say those words. Ready? Bat...cat...hat. Again. Bat...cat...hat. *Continue this procedure with other rhymes. Give clues for the children to identify a third rhyming word for each pair. Suggestions:*

    me - bee - tree
    hop - top - drop
    tug - bug - rug
    rake - cake - snake
    goat - boat - coat

    Recommendation: Allow children to suggest nonsense words that rhyme. If they suggest words that do not rhyme, point out the error. Explain why the two words the child provided do not rhyme, then suggest possible rhyming word pairs.

7. I have a rhyme to share. Listen very carefully. *Repeat the first two lines of a rhyme, such as "Little Boy Blue." Emphasize the words that rhyme ("horn" and "corn"). Say:* In this rhyme "horn" and "corn" are two words that sound like each other. "Horn" and "corn" are called rhyming words because they have the same ending sounds. Now, you say them with me, and listen to their sounds. Horn...corn. Again. Horn...corn. Now, let's repeat the rhyme *(emphasize italicized words):*

    Little Boy Blue, come blow your *horn.*
    The sheep's in the meadow; the cow's in the *corn...*

8. Listen carefully as I say two words that rhyme. "Run"..."gun." Again. "Run"..."gun." They both end with the "un" sound. Now, you say them. Ready? Run...gun. Again. Run...gun. Can you think of something to put a hamburger on that rhymes with "run" and "gun?" Yes, it is "bun." Let's say those three words. Ready? Run...gun...bun.

9. I have some sentences to share with you. But, I need your help. I want you to finish them for me by telling me words that rhyme. Ready? *Suggestions:*

    The old black cat is wearing a ________________.
    The little brown mouse lives in a ________________.
    The sly old fox climbed into a ________________.
    The mean old goat ate my ________________.

10. I have a rhyme to share. Listen very carefully. *Repeat the first two lines of a rhyme, such as "Humpty Dumpty." Emphasize the words that rhyme ("wall" and "fall"). Say:* In this rhyme "wall" and "fall" are two words that sound like each other. "Wall" and "fall" are called rhyming words because they have the same ending sounds. Now, you say them with me, and listen to their sounds. Wall...fall. Again. Wall...fall. Now, let's repeat the rhyme *(emphasize italicized words):*

    Humpty Dumpty sat on a *wall.*
    Humpty Dumpty had a great *fall...*

11. *Display two pictures of objects that are not rhyming words (such as "mouse" and "tree"). Ask children to name the pictures. Then ask:* Can you find the picture that rhymes with "bee?" *Continue with other pictures, displaying two pictures that do not rhyme at a time. Ask each child to participate. If a child names a word that does not rhyme, explain why the two do not rhyme, and help the child say a word that does rhyme. Repeat this activity several times.*

12. *Display one picture (such as "tree"). Ask children to name the picture, then ask:* Can you think of a word that rhymes with "tree?" *Continue to display other pictures, asking children to name a word that rhymes with each. Be sure to give each child an opportunity to participate. If a child names a word that does not rhyme with the stimulus word, explain why the two words do not rhyme.*

Materials: Five pairs of pictures of objects that rhyme ("tree" and "bee," "house" and "mouse," "sock" and "clock," "ball" and "wall," "car" and "star")
Large bag

13. *Display one picture of each rhyming pair. Place the matching pairs in the bag. Say:* Please choose one picture from the bag. Tell what it is. Then, find the rhyming picture on the table, and put the two rhyming pictures together in front of you. *Ask each child to participate. Repeat the activity several times.*

14. *Place pairs of pictures face down in front of the children. Say:* Let's play "Memory." Turn two pictures over. If they rhyme, you get to keep them. If they do not rhyme, turn them back over, and the next person will play. *Ask each child to participate in turn.*

15. *Display three pictures (two that rhyme and one that does not). Ask children to name all three pictures. Then say:* Find the two pictures that rhyme. *Continue with other sets of three pictures, displaying two rhyming and one nonrhyming picture each time. Ask children to identify the two pictures that rhyme. Make sure each child participates. Repeat activity several times.*

    Repeat this activity, increasing the number of pictures displayed to four (two rhyming, two nonrhyming).

PROGRESS CHECK

Materials: None

Listen carefully. I am going to say three words that rhyme or do not rhyme. If the words I say rhyme, you say, "Yes." If the words do not rhyme, say, "No." Let's try. Top...cop...pop. Yes, all three of these words rhyme. Let's try again. Grow...pet...toe. No, all these words do not rhyme.

When you are certain the child understands the task, say the following groups of words:

frog - dog -log
brown - town - corn
fall - wall - hall
corn - horn - born
tree - bee- hill

Scoring:

+	Responds correctly to all five sets of words, with no prompts
0	Fails to respond correctly to all five pairs, requiring more than one prompt

Index of Illustrations

LILAC

The End